DISCARD

Machines in Medicine

Other Books in this Series

Machines in Medicine

The Medical Practice of the Future

Donald Longmore

Edited and Illustrated
by M. Ross-Macdonald

Doubleday Science Series
Doubleday & Company, Inc.
Garden City, New York, 1970

610.72
L856

First published in the United States of America in 1970 by Doubleday
& Company, Inc., Garden City, New York, in association with
Aldus Books Limited
Library of Congress Catalog Card No. 73-79647
Printed in Italy by Arnoldo Mondadori, Verona

Contents

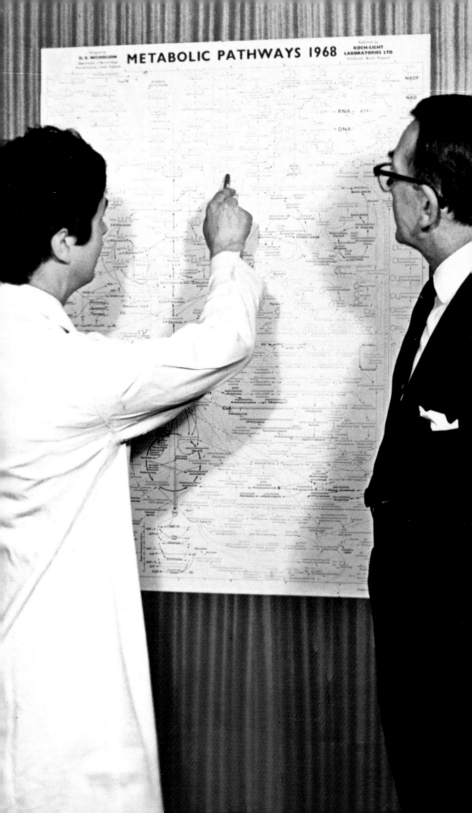

METABOLIC PATHWAYS 1968

1 The Cell, The Organ, The Organism

Few doctors have ever seen the most important machines in medicine: scanning electron microscopes that can show, in shallow relief, living cells at work, enlarged hundreds of thousands of times; microscopic dissection apparatus that can peel the cell apart; ultracentrifuges that can separate minute cellular components; microelectrodes that measure potential differences across membranes only a few molecules thick; chromatographs and isotope counters that can analyze the contents of droplets as small as 10^{-4} cc.—just visible to a good eye. Indeed, most doctors would not classify these devices as medical machines at all. Yet the fact remains that fundamental progress in medicine now rests with these machines, all of which have one common feature: we use them to unravel the complex processes within living cells, and their myriad interactions with one another. By contrast, the machines that most people would call "medical" operate at the most gross statistical level; they sum one or two aspects of the function of millions of specialized cells; and from these clues we hopefully "diagnose" and with the aid of equally crude devices

A biochemist and a doctor confer over the probable site of failure in a vital pathway of the cell's metabolism. The difficulties of understanding and curing disease at this level and the important part that bio-engineering must play in medicine are fully discussed in this chapter.

we hopefully "treat" the sick bodies and minds that come within our scrutiny.

The practice of medicine has always been confined by the available machinery. Open-heart surgery, for instance, was possible in the 1930s but for the lack of two machines: a heart-lung machine to take over the pumping and gas-exchange functions, and a machine to extract and purify the anti-clotting factor *heparin* from animals' blood. (Without an increased amount of heparin the patient's blood would clot on the foreign surfaces of the heart-lung machine.) All the machines routinely used by doctors and specialists work at this organic, or whole-body, level. The amazing thing is not that our success has been so modest, but that we have had any success at all. For the seat of most disease lies inside the living cell—in regions that machines never directly reach (except by the crude, sledgehammer techniques of X-ray bombardment).

True, we do have ways of influencing intracellular activity. We can put into the blood synthetic hormones, or simple salts used in normal metabolism, or antibiotics extracted from mold cultures. But the purpose is always to allow some natural cellular process to reassert itself; we are not directly engineering the cell's functional anatomy so that distorted processes resume normal patterns. To make this point clear let me frame the sort of question that I imagine medical students will be answering in their finals in the year 2000 or so. It runs as follows:

"A patient is referred to you as suffering from anxiety, which preliminary examination has shown is due to an excess of lactate. The cause, however, is not the usual locking of the membrane calcium carriers but an inhibition of the Krebs cycle by the substance whose structure is shown on your console. It is, as you see, a mismade enzyme. Identify the true enzyme and either (i) say how you would restructure the patient's DNA so as to correct the synthesis, or (ii) design a blocking molecule to inhibit the mismade enzyme (only 20 per cent of the patient's production of this enzyme takes this mismade form). In either case, give the carrier pathway into the cell for the molecule you design. (Central computer time 10 minutes; personal computer time 30 minutes.)"

The student who successfully answers such questions will be

both doctor and molecular engineer. And the machines I mentioned at the outset will be part of his discipline. They will be medical machines. If you are alive in the year 2000, and some publisher of that era brings out a book with the same title as this one, what unimaginable riches of *real* knowledge will lie waiting between its covers! You will look back on this book as we now look back on medieval alchemy—as a hotch-potch of half-digested facts and misapplied thought. There is, however, one vital difference: alchemists believed they were on the right track; we know we are, if not on the wrong track, at least on one whose goals are inadequate. Our problem, basically, is the impossibility of designing machines that in any way match the subtlety of living matter. We appreciate the inadequacy and we know that it is forced upon us by a secondhand technology—the crumbs from the tables of other branches of science and engineering.

By way of encouragement I will add that I do not intend to write the whole book in this negative tone—which is really why I began it that way. When I later enthuse about some machine or other and point to its elaborate ingenuity (or to its beautiful simplicity) my enthusiasm is relative—based in the 1960s. You must add the longer perspective that I am about to outline.

We begin by looking at the general nature of cellular activity and then consider the boundary between the machines we use and organisms composed of such cells.

A Portrait of the Cell

There is no typical cell; but if we eliminate all the features related to specialized functions (such as hemoglobin in red blood cells, or the specialized membranes of kidney cells) we can paint a fairly clear elementary portrait of the features that allow a cell to exist, manufacture substances, imbibe, digest, and excrete. We are looking for active principles, so the anatomy will be functional and the details highly generalized.

Such a generalized portrait appears on page 13. The two chief features are the outer membrane, which marks the boundary of the cell, and the nucleus, which directs its activity. Between them is the *cytoplasm*, which contains a number of defined structures known as *organelles*.

The *nucleus* contains the cell's DNA (deoxyribonucleic acid), which is, in effect, a blueprint that determines the cell's structure and function. Barring mutation here and there, every nucleus in our body contains identical DNA—that is, all the information needed to re-create us is contained in each one of our cells. Clearly, since each specialized cell performs only one function out of the myriads of possible bodily functions, most of the DNA is somehow "switched off." Only the part that controls the cell in question and regulates its specific function is activated. Between cell divisions the DNA is contained by the *chromatin strands*, which are spread loosely within the nucleus. Just before division these coil up into tight strands—the *chromosomes*. At the same time the *centriole* divides into two daughter centrioles, which act as the poles of the axis along which first the chromosomes and then the nucleus divide.

The *ribosomes*, which cluster around the *endoplasmic reticulum*, are sites of protein manufacture. The reticulum is, in effect, a deep and convoluted invagination of the outer membrane, which brings extracellular material into the innermost parts of the cell—even to the nuclear membrane itself. The exact mechanism of protein synthesis is outside the scope of this present survey (but see Suggested Reading). It is enough to note that a cell rich in endoplasmic reticulum and ribosomes is heavily engaged in protein synthesis; a cell poor in these organelles is merely ticking over, as far as protein output goes. The *Golgi apparatus*, continuous with the endoplasmic reticulum, is smooth-membraned and devoid of ribosomes. It acts as a parceling depot for secretions from the reticulum (and perhaps elsewhere). The secretions lodge in small recesses, where they grow by addition until they are large enough to leave the main apparatus and, wrapped in smooth membrane, make their way to the outer wall. There they pass outside, rupture, and release their contents.

The *nucleolus* performs the same function for the nucleus as the ribosomes perform for the cell in general—it manufactures nuclear protein. The *lysosome* is a kind of "poisons cupboard" within the cell. It contains *enzymes* (protein-like catalysts) that are needed in digestion of food but that, if they were diffused throughout the cell, would digest the cell instead. The lysosomal

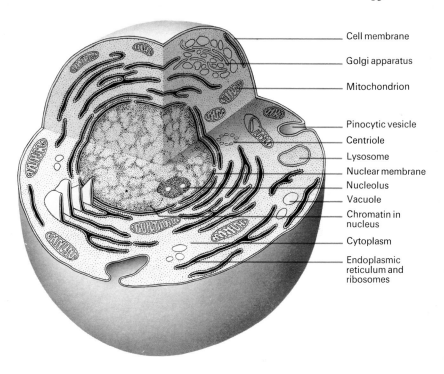

Cell membrane

Golgi apparatus

Mitochondrion

Pinocytic vesicle

Centriole

Lysosome

Nuclear membrane

Nucleolus

Vacuole

Chromatin in nucleus

Cytoplasm

Endoplasmic reticulum and ribosomes

The diagram shows a typical cell and its parts—all discussed in the text. The size and contrast of the organelles are exaggerated for the sake of clarity. The electron micrograph (right) shows the double-layered structure of the cell membrane (× 46,000).

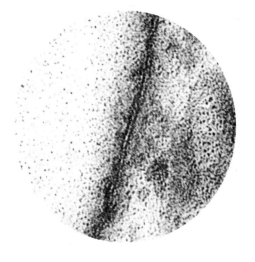

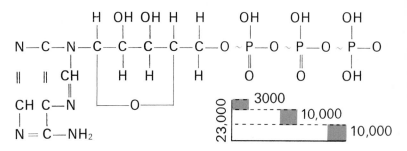

Structural formula of ATP molecule shows, in color, the three energy-rich phosphate bonds. Removal of final phosphate group (right) turns ATP to ADP (diphosphate), the bond yielding 10,000 calories per mole (gram molecular weight) of ATP. Removal of penultimate phosphate group turns ADP to AMP (monophosphate), again yielding 10,000 calories per mole of ATP. Removal of remaining phosphate group creates plain adenosine, yielding 3000 calories per mole of the original ATP. To reconstruct ATP from ADP, AMP, or adenosine requires an equivalent amount of energy.

membrane isolates these enzymes from the rest of the cell. When they are needed they are transported in small quantities through the membrane and ferried in some kind of inactive state until they reach the macromolecules of protein, fat, and nucleic acid, which it is their job to break down. The broken remnants of these macromolecules are processed in the *mitochondria*. These are minute sausage-shaped structures with twin membranes. Like the endoplasmic reticulum, the inner membrane is deeply involuted, forming sacs called *cristae*. On the inner surfaces of the cristae are protein complexes bathed in oxidative enzymes. The breakdown products of digestion, transported through the outer membrane, are here oxidized, yielding up the energy stored in their chemical bonds to energy-carrying molecules in the cell—chief among them being adenosine triphosphate (ATP). Wandering freely through the cell, ATP can arrive at any one of thousands of sites and give up energy by turning into a lower-energy molecule— ADP (diphosphate), AMP (monophosphate), or just plain adenosine. The adenosine and the free phosphate groups can be rebuilt to ATP by the energy-yielding processes of metabolism; the rebuilding is chiefly associated with the mitochondria—often called the "powerhouses" of living cells.

The *pinocytic* and *phagocytic vesicles* are ad hoc involutions of the cell membrane—a system for engulfing liquid and solid raw materials respectively, from the extracellular medium. When the involution runs deep enough into the cell, it pinches off at the neck, creating a vacuole. Because the vacuole is surrounded by membrane, it is, in the amorphous topology of the cell, "outside" the system. Material from it is transported into the cell by mechanisms identical with those in the cell's outer membrane.

Membranes

One word has repeatedly cropped up throughout this brief outline of the cell: *membrane*. These skins around the cell and its organelles are no mere passive barriers that prevent the cell's contents from spilling out; they play a very active role in passing substances into and out of the cell. These transport mechanisms, which are still poorly understood, will one day provide the key to much that is mysterious about the cell's activity.

The typical cell membrane has been likened to a bread-and-butter sandwich—an affinity for fat in the middle, an affinity for water at the outsides. Its structural elements are fatty molecules known as *phospholipids* (see diagram on page 17). They contain two fatty-acid chains attached to a glycerol molecule (the fat-soluble end) to which is attached one of a number of phosphate-containing molecules (the water-soluble end). One must not think of these as permanent bricks in the cell wall; in response to information from both inside and outside the cell, they can change form (that is, change from one phospholipid to another) instantaneously. Moreover they are coated with sheets and globules o protein and enzymes.

This sandwich is not uniform over the whole membrane surface. About one thousandth of its area is taken up by minute pores—too small to show in an electron micrograph but large enough to allow metallic ions, water, and other small molecules through. These pores allow the elementary transport mechanisms of osmosis, solvent drag, and electric potential gradient to operate (see diagrams on page 18). The tendency of these mechanisms is to produce equilibrium on each side of the membrane. Cells, however, need to be in constant disequilibrium with their surroundings; otherwise they die. For instance, cells are rich in large molecules; the fluid that bathes them is relatively poor. There is thus an endless tendency for water to invade the cell to equalize the concentration. If this tendency were not checked, cells would swell, rupture, and die. The histogram on page 20 shows the concentrations of the various solutes in the body fluids. The measure is given in milliequivalents (mEq.) rather than in the more familiar millimoles because most body solutes are, in solution, split up into separate ions. The effectiveness of these ions in the chemical reactions of metabolism depends upon the number of positive or negative charges they carry, i.e. upon their valency. Thus, substances like Ca^{++} are twice as effective as Na^+ in mopping up, for instance, HCO_3^-. Effective concentrations are measured in terms of equivalents, determined by dividing the atomic weight of a substance by its valency. The atomic weight of calcium is 40 and its gram equivalent weight is thus $40/2 = 20$ gm. A milliequivalent of calcium is, of course, a thousandth part of 20 gm.

Almost all animal cells respond to this threat by pumping out sodium ions, so that their concentration outside may be 50 times the internal concentration; this evens out the osmotic forces. It also creates an electrical potential of about one tenth of a volt—which, across a membrane only one millionth of a centimeter thick, is no mean force. These potential differences are important in nerve impulses and muscular contractions.

So, in contrast to the passive transport of substances through the pores, the membrane actively transports substances out of the cell against fairly hefty gradients of concentration and electrical potential. The cell expends a good proportion of its energy in this one function. The exact mechanism is still unknown, although it seems to involve changes in configuration of the phospholipid molecules. The energy for these changes comes from ATP, synthesized in the mitochondria. Furthermore, fresh phospholipids are constantly manufactured within the cytoplasm. Thus, although the phenomenon of active transport occurs at the membrane, the inner recesses of the cell play a fully committed role in maintaining it. In Chapter 4 we shall look at the mechanisms that maintain the gradients against which the membranes work.

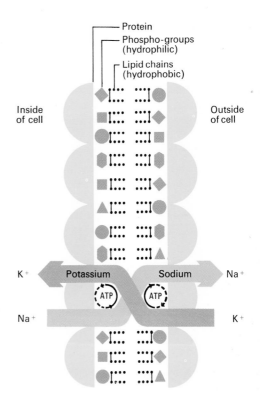

Schematized structure of membrane and model of the Na⁺/K⁺ ion pump are shown. The membrane is discussed at length in the text. The two phospholipid layers are impermeable to ions, but combined with a carrier molecule the ions can pass through easily. The energy for such active transport is provided by the conversion of ATP to ADP.

Why does the cell go to such lengths to maintain this external-internal imbalance? In answering this question we come close to the nature of life itself. Life is characterized by highly unlikely concentrations of macromolecules, rich in energy, diverse in shape, and capable of multiple bonds with other such molecules. When these molecules are temporarily bonded, they alter their configurations. Such alterations change their ability to interact, so that divergent chemical pathways temporarily converge, leading to reactions and products unknown elsewhere in the universe. The proteins that mediate such temporary linkups (they are called *allosteric* enzymes) closely resemble the components of electrical networks, in that they select from, amplify, regulate, accelerate, or damp down the input and the products. In short, it is by no means fanciful to talk of the cell as a microcosm, a densely packed information-handling system. At any moment the cell has the ability to select from the entire genetic information just the part that relates to the needs created by internal and external conditions. The macromolecules that do the selecting are identical with those that communicate the structural information, regulate synthesis, and perform all the other cellular functions. This tightly knit community simply loses the ability to function when its members are pushed apart and set adrift in an ocean of ions, water molecules, and other small compounds. The membrane is all that stands between this community and such chaos.

The Organ and the Organism

It is this kind of complexity that we should bear in mind as we try to adapt this picture of the generalized cell. ("Picture" is a most inadequate word; the macromolecules I mentioned can interact a thousand times a second—we are obviously "picturing"

Passive transport mechanisms (so called because they consume no energy) are diagramed below. In osmosis the large solute molecules (orange) attract the smaller solvent molecules through pores in the membrane and the cell tends to swell until equilibrium is reached. Inrushing solvent molecules can drag in solute molecules with them, causing solvent drag. If positive and negative ions are unevenly distributed, they too will move through the pores until the potential gradient is abolished. By actively exporting positive ions, in the form of Na+, the cell sets up a potential gradient in opposition to the osmotic gradient, thus ensuring a greater solute concentration within.

Osmosis   Solvent drag   Potential gradient events in highly cerebral terms, far above the level of any animated diagram.) Think of our cell as a primitive member of that tiny embryonic colony that in nine months will become a viable human organism. Imagine it dividing every eight hours; imbibing amino acids, sugars, fats, minerals, oxygen, vitamins, hormones, enzymes; making new protein, new membrane, new DNA; excreting wastes, CO_2, hormones, enzymes; regulating the other cells in the embryo, and being regulated by them. Think of its ever-swelling progeny slowly turning into specialized cells—muscle, blood, nerve, cartilage. As the process goes on, picture the endless interchange of secretions that regulate the timing and evenness of this phenomenal growth and specialization. Imagine their effect on each cell's DNA—switching parts off here, parts on there, permanently in one kind of cell, temporarily in another. Think of how the cells respond: one takes up more glycogen, another more amino acid, another ceases to grow, another withers and dies.

Do you still have any kind of picture? No, of course not. We can just about conceive the operation of a single transport activity in the membrane of one cell. The ordered jostling of giant molecules within the cell is beyond our conceptual power. We could more easily map and chronicle the story of Man—giving every kinship, every life story of every man and woman who ever lived, every minor detail of every dwelling, farmstead, street, and city that ever was—than we could conceive of the activity within a three-month-old embryo. And yet in this picture I am attempting to sketch we are only just arriving at the level on which the most elegant medical machines operate—machines that communicate with the body via a handful of electrodes, a few tubes, a bunch of sensors.

The user of such machines is in a curious position, analogous to that of the China-watcher in politics. There is a country seething with revolution and counter-revolution, undergoing enormous industrial expansion (or is it stagnation?), its agriculture taking great leaps forward (or backward?), tightly controlled from the center (or is that a fiction?)—a country that is sealed off from the kind of investigation we can make in any other part of the world. And there sits the China-watcher, surrounded by his electronic

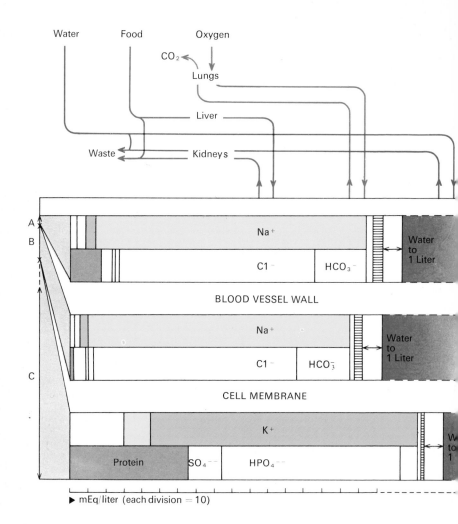

Water   Food   Oxygen

CO_2

Lungs

Liver

Waste   Kidneys

A
B

Na^+

Water to 1 Liter

Cl^- HCO_3^-

BLOOD VESSEL WALL

Na^+

Water to 1 Liter

Cl^- HCO_3^-

CELL MEMBRANE

C

K^+

W to 1

Protein SO_4^{--} HPO_4^{--}

▶ mEq/liter (each division = 10)

This schematic view of metabolism emphasizes the body fluids and their electrolytes (nonelectrolyte solutes are shown hatched). The relative quantities of body fluids typical for a 70-kg. adult are shown at left. A represents blood serum (3 liters); B represents interstitial fluid (9 liters); and C represents cell fluid (30-35 liters). Note that the cell fluid (lower bar) is richer in solutes than the interstitial fluid (middle bar) that bathes the cell, thus creating an osmotic gradient against which the cell must constantly export Na^+ ions (see text). Unlabeled constituents include ionic magnesium, calcium, potassium, organic acid, sulfate, phosphate, carbonic acid, and various nonelectrolytes. Two-way arrows at ends of bars indicate normal variation.

listening apparatus and his press clippings—to get information from *them* he must stand logic on its head. For the rest he relies on minute clues—tales told by escapees, snippets of party documents that fall into the wrong hands. From such minutiae he must make the kind of assessment that is difficult to make in even the most open society. It isn't that nothing is happening in China; it isn't that he lacks elaborate watching and measuring devices; it is that the channels between observer and observed are so thin that the information that struggles through them is distorted before it begins and out of date when it arrives. Medical machinery has exactly the same characteristics. The machinery may be as elaborate as human ingenuity can make it; and the body's activity is certainly elaborate beyond our finest conceptual power; but the channel that links the two—their interface—is incommensurably narrow.

The Interface

Because medical machines are designed to fit the organism, and not vice versa, we can classify the interface in terms of organic activity—chemical, electrical, and mechanical. The following chapters examine these categories in greater detail. So let me close this general survey with a few general remarks, which will also serve as an introduction to more detailed analysis.

Whatever their precise nature, all interfaces are, in effect, crude "summing junctions." They measure the results or products of billions of reactions within the body. Perhaps a further analogy will help to make this clear. To take a blood sample from a person and to infer from it what is happening in his cells is like trying to discover a city's industrial activity from samples of its effluents and atmospheric pollution. How is it that any useful information emerges? The key lies in the fact that cellular behavior is *determined*. An external influence that affects one cell is capable of affecting all other cells of the same type. When such influences extend to large cell populations, the results begin to show at the coarse levels that come within the resolving power, so to speak, of the body-machine interface. Nobody notices the loss of a few hundred nerve cells, or even of hundreds of millions of red corpuscles, but when enough such cells are lost for the result to show—as a local paralysis, for example, or in reduced heart function—then we begin to get useful information through the interface.

This explains why single measurements, or even a string of measurements of a single function, are seldom enough to produce an accurate diagnosis, especially now that our powers to intervene in disorders and reverse their course are growing. For example, I know of a cardiac specialist who, while dancing fairly energetically with a nurse at a hospital ball, correctly diagnosed an incipient but serious heart condition. The information was of the simplest kind—the color of her lips, the pattern of her breathing, and a brief snatch of her pulse. Not so long ago there was little he could have done—a few drugs and a bit of advice. Curing her condition would have involved opening the heart and an artery, replacing certain parts, and sewing her up again—all of which was then impossible. In such circumstances the kind of diagnosis he made (confirmed in more orthodox surroundings, of course) would have been enough. As it happened, the girl's condition was operable. The risks were slight, but real enough to call for more detailed investigation before we attempted any surgery. So before she came near the operating theater we took electrocardiograms (EKG's), angiograms, and lung-function tests, and we physically examined the defect by working a catheter up an artery in her arm until it reached the site of the trouble. If her case had been an emergency one, any of these measurements of the heart and nearby vessels would have been enough to justify the operation. But since there was no urgency, we wanted to be as informed as possible about her defect. So we had to combine scant information from a whole series of tests and to interpret each in the light of the others.

To restate these last three sentences in the more general terms of information theory: data through a single channel may be marred by error and drowned by noise, but by getting the same data in different forms through a number of channels we automatically achieve an elementary noise filter and an error-correcting code. In every field of medicine where machines are involved, this channel-duplication technique is providing a powerful means of compensating for the fundamental inadequacy of the interface.

Even so, all the duplication in the world will not overcome that inadequacy. The nurse's heart defect, for instance, was congenital. Its roots lay in her embryonic past: due either to a misreading of the genetic code or to a mistiming of its application. The nurse is now healthier than she ever was before the operation, but the proper way to treat such defects would be to prevent them from happening in the first place, not to let them mess up a person's youth and adolescence, and certainly not to let them get so serious that their effects outweigh the risks of major surgery. From all that I have said in this chapter you can imagine how far off this ultimate therapy still lies.

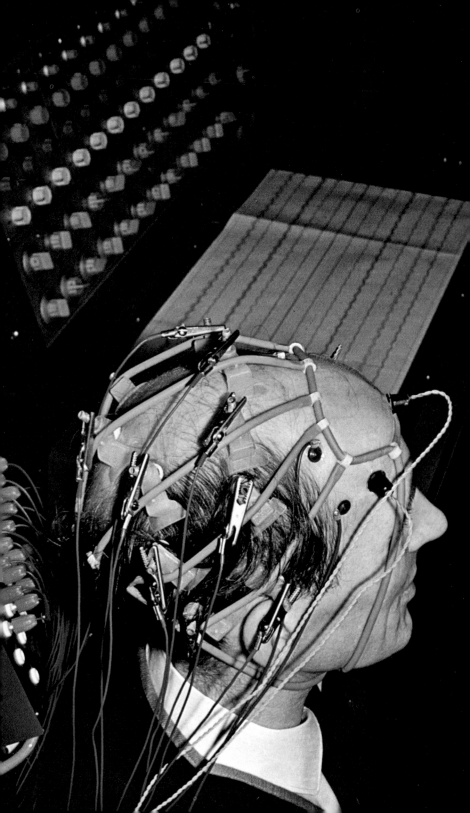

2 Measuring Electrical Activity

One of the most important functions for all medical machines is measurement. This is, by definition, true of diagnostic machinery. It is also, though less obviously, true of machines used in therapy or for temporary support; for instance, we need to measure the body's response to the inputs from the machine. Broadly speaking, the measurements we make fall into three categories: electrical (measurements of nerve and muscle function), chemical (measurements of bodily metabolism), and mechanical (measurements of movements, capacities, and throughputs). Let us start by looking at the nature of this information—how it arises and how it gets to the interface. In this chapter we are concerned with electrical information—taking EEG's (electroencephalographs) and EKG's (electrocardiographs) as examples. Later chapters will consider the other categories.

Our nervous system contains just over 10^{10} nerve cells, most of which are in the brain; the remainder are very unevenly distributed throughout the body. Our eyes, for instance, contain over 250 million receptors. The center of the spleen is practically

Recording brain waves is perhaps the most familiar measurement of the body's electrical activity. Extremely sensitive and reliable machines have been devised but interpretation of the results still demands very special care. The patient in this picture is fitted with three types of electrodes. The rubber suction caps on the forehead are filled with electrode jelly and electrical contact is made through this by a pure silver pole. The pure silver/silver chloride disk electrodes behind these are very reliable and especially suitable for sleep recordings and for children. The pad electrodes, which are held in place by the rubber harness, are widely used for initial screening of patients.

nerveless. Yet, as in any communications system, the truly remarkable feature of this network is not its multiplicity of channels but the richness of their interconnection. Each brain cell is estimated to connect with between 5000 and 50,000 other brain cells. Even the lower figure—10^{10} cells each with 5000 connections—gives a network of astronomical dimensions, quite beyond its own ability to comprehend itself. Fortunately other parts of the network have simpler structures more fitted to their humbler roles. Even here, though, the richness of interconnection is still vital.

The Nerve Impulse

The diagram on this page shows the reflex that produces a knee jerk when the tendon below the kneecap is sharply stretched. It consists of two kinds of receptor and one effector. (In reality hundreds of such nerves are involved, but the principle can be illustrated with one of each category.) The effector is a *motor neuron*, a cell with its nucleus in the spinal cord and a long fiber reaching down to a thigh muscle. The sensory nerves are of two kinds—*excitatory* and *inhibitory*; the excitatory fiber acts directly upon the motor neuron, causing it to "fire"; the inhibitory fiber

Network responsible for starting and halting the knee-jerk reflex is diagramed below. When the tendon below the knee is tapped, stretch receptors (A) in muscles on the front of the thigh are stretched. Nerve impulses set up in such receptors trigger excitation in the motor neuron body, causing these muscles to contract. However, opposing muscles on the rear of the thigh are stretched, and receptors (B) in these muscles stimulate the inhibitory neuron, which prevents further excitations in the motor neuron. In all skeletal muscle this opposition of excitation and inhibition plays a central part in maintaining smooth movement and in checking excesses.

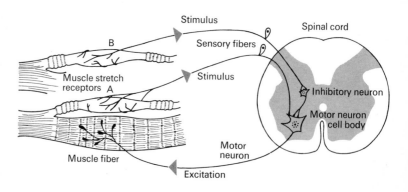

acts through an *inhibitory neuron*, which can inhibit the firing sequence.

At first sight it may seem strange that the network has this built-in opposition of excitation and inhibition. The explanation lies in the nature of the nervous impulse itself, which is a binary phenomenon—that is, a fiber either fires or it doesn't; there is no in-between state.

The membrane around the fiber employs the sodium pump described in the previous chapter (see diagram on page 17). It pumps Na^+ (sodium) ions outward so that the outside concentration is about 10 times the inside concentration. On the "return stroke," so to speak, it pumps K^+ (potassium) ions inward so that there are 30 times as many potassium ions inside as outside. But the total quantities of potassium are much lower than those of sodium, so there is a net positive charge on the outside of about +70 millivolts (a millivolt is a thousandth of a volt). In other words the membrane is polarized; when a nerve is stimulated, pores in the membrane open, allowing the Na^+ ions to flood inward and so reverse the electrical polarity. In less than a millisecond the polarity reaches +30 millivolts inside and then the outward flow of K^+ ions (which hitherto were held by the same

The nerve impulse. In the unstimulated fiber the sodium pump maintains an unequal distribution of Na^+ and K^+ ions across the membrane, resulting in a resting potential. When stimulated a small region of the membrane becomes permeable to Na^+ ions. The sudden reversal of charge produced by the inrush of Na^+ ions generates cyclic electric currents that cause corresponding permeability changes as they pass along the membrane. This moving wave of depolarization is the nerve impulse. Following its passage the original polarity is partly restored by an outflow of K^+ ions and then the membrane becomes repolarized as Na^+ and K^+ ions resume their former concentrations.

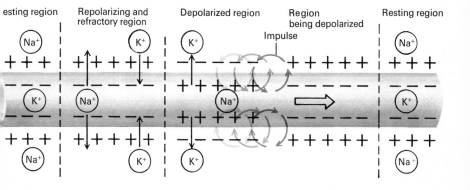

forces that caused the inrush of Na^+ ions) partly restores the original polarity. The Na-K pumps do the rest. This reversal of polarization passes like a wave down the fiber (see the diagram on the previous page).

In effect, a nerve with its polarity at the full 70 millivolts is like a loaded gun with a hair trigger—a highly unstable system. The instability accounts for the speed at which nerve impulses travel—up to 300 meters per second. It also accounts for the two built-in safeguards—the inhibitory neurons, and the fact that many incoming excitations are needed to fire a single motor neuron.

Disappointingly enough, with two exceptions, we have no way of measuring these impulses at the skin. No doubt they do arrive at the skin, but by then they are so attenuated as to be drowned in the general background of electrical activity from the muscles. The two exceptions are the brain and the neck, where we can measure the activity of the phrenic nerve. This nerve relays impulses between the hindbrain and the diaphragm. Our ability to measure its activity is not as useful as you might think, for we have no way of discriminating the direction of the nerve impulse. A burst of phrenic nerve activity on the chart or scope may be an upward train of information about the position of the diaphragm or a downward train of impulses to regulate that position. With the electrical patterns of the brain it is quite a different story.

The Electroencephalograph

Pairs of exploring electrodes placed at various points on the exposed brain will record potential differences of between 30 and 600 microvolts (millionths of a volt). Similar electrodes on the scalp usually record differences up to only 200 microvolts. In other words, the minute electrical changes that occur on the brain surface are attenuated to about a third of their original strength by the intervening centimeter of fluid, bone, skin, and hair. If we explore the scalp systematically, we soon notice that in each region the potentials fluctuate rhythmically, and that the frequencies are characteristically slowest near the forehead, quicker above the ears, quicker still at the back, and quickest of all at the top (see diagram opposite).

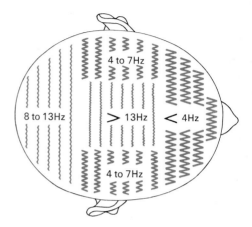

Characteristic output frequencies of EEG waves in various regions of the scalp (1 Hz.= 1 cycle per second).

No one knows how these brain waves are produced, though it is almost certain that they arise in the huge nerve populations of the fore- and midbrain (which together make up the bulk of the brain), and that the two regions interact. All our clinical experience of these waves is thus empirical rather than based on sound theory: we know that certain patterns are signs of abnormality but we do not know why they should take a particular form.

The electrodes most widely used are silver disks held in place by collodion or adhesive caps, as shown on page 24. To ensure good electrical contact the operator parts the hair and rubs the scalp with a light abrasive; this removes fats, oils, and dead skin—all nonconductors. He then puts a conducting jelly between the electrode and the scalp. If the resistance is higher than 5000 ohms, good recording is impossible.

The drawing on page 30 shows the standard electrode positions for routine examination; how many positions are used in any given session depends on the number of recording channels in the electroencephalograph. Some have only 2 channels, others more than 16, but 8-channel machines are the commonest, because they are just within the range of easy portability, which is important when the patient cannot be moved. As with the EKG, the experts are always asking for more channels; but many observations can be made quite simply from only 2 channels. In the operating theater, for instance, where rhythm changes are

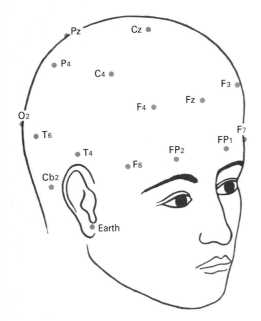

Left: internationally recognized positions for EEG electrodes. All points except those on the mid-line (Pz, Cz, and Fz) are symmetrical with similar points on the left side of the head (e.g. FP₁ and FP₂). Below and opposite: seven standard EEG montages for recording on an 8-channel machine.

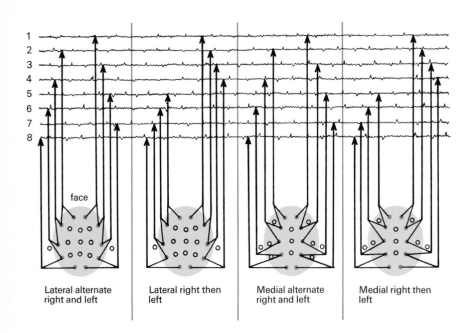

Lateral alternate right and left

Lateral right then left

Medial alternate right and left

Medial right then left

muscles. The stripes are caused by the regular interleaving of two kinds of protein fiber, *actin* and *myosin*, which make up the bulk of the muscle and give it the ability to move rapidly.

The interleaving of actin and myosin is sketched on page 36, where the contractile sequence is also shown. The actin filament is a double helix of globular proteins; the myosin filament is composed of match-like proteins arranged down its long axis and with their "heads" (globular fractions) away from the central region. It is the movement of the actin filaments over the globules of the myosin filaments that constitutes muscular movement—not a coiling-up process in these proteins. The actin filaments are drawn in between the myosin filaments by a ratchet-like mechanism involving the alternate making and breaking of bridges between the globular regions of the myosin molecules and active sites on the actin filaments. Evidence suggests that the myosin heads actually constitute the cross bridges and that these regions also contain the necessary ATP-splitting enzymes.

Unlike many other tissues, muscles do not possess well-defined cells. In the embryo, muscles arise from the fusion of cells called *myoblasts*. The fused cells (called *myofibrils*) develop regular bands of actin and myosin and grow a common membrane called the *sarcolemma*. In the resting state the electrical potential outside the sarcolemma is about 100 millivolts above that of the inside. The sarcolemma maintains this potential by pumping out calcium ions against the electrical gradient. In the negatively charged internal environment the energy necessary to build the temporary actin-myosin bridges cannot be released. But as soon as the depolarization wave arrives from the nerve, it triggers a similarly rapid wave along the sarcolemma, changing it in some way that allows Ca^{++} ions to flood inward. The opening is very brief, for the original polarization is restored in a fraction of a second. Nevertheless this brief reversal is long enough to allow enzymes within the myofibril to split ATP and so release energy to build the actin-myosin bridges.

A muscle 10 cm. thick contains in cross section some 10 million myofibrils. The electrical impulse we can pick up at the skin is the collective and almost instantaneous depolarization of some

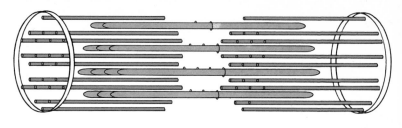

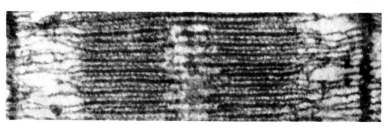

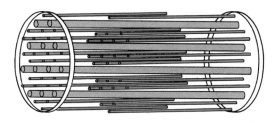

Interleafing of actin (red) and myosin (gray) in relaxed muscle fibers is shown at top. The electron micrograph shows part of a corresponding section of striated muscle. Muscular contraction involves the sliding of actin filaments in between the myosin filaments until, at full contraction, the actin filaments overlap as shown above. The myosin filament is about 1.5 microns long.

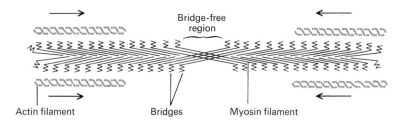

Contact between actin and myosin is represented above. The myosin filament consists of myosin molecules with their heads (zigzag lines) pointing away from the central region. These extend as cross-bridges to active sites on the actin filament, and by changing shape they move the actin filaments along the myosin filament—a make-and-break ratchet mechanism.

of this vast array. When the effort is slight, only a few of the myofibrils are depolarizing at any given moment; when it is severe, most of them are. The maximum depolarization of our greatest muscle—the quadriceps in the thigh—creates electrical variations at the nearest point to the skin of only a couple of millivolts.

The fact that depolarization and repolarization in deep-lying muscles creates electrical variations at the skin is the basis of a whole group of medical machines. In my earlier book I described how such variations can be used as signals to control pacemakers, prosthetic limbs, or machine tools; they can also be used for diagnosis—as in the electrocardiograph (EKG).

The Electrocardiograph

Contrary to widespread belief, the EKG does not actually measure the muscular activity of the heart—we can, in fact, get a normal electrical reading from a heart that has ceased to beat. The energy that moves the recording pen (or flying spot of electrons on an oscilloscope) derives from the inward and outward flow of ions through the membranes of the heart muscle. These flows invariably precede the muscular contraction and relaxation, so that the membrane has depolarized and even begun to repolarize before the muscle begins to move. But the change in polarization only makes muscle action *possible*; it does not guarantee it.

The path of this de- and repolarization wave through the heart is shown on page 38. If we peppered the heart with electrodes we could measure the waves flowing along each of the many directions shown, but because the heart is accessible only in major surgery, we are usually confined to readings between two poles or to readings from single electrodes placed at various points around the chest. Thus the EKG is a measure of the resultant of all the waves moving through the heart at any given moment. The same diagram shows how two waves, traveling along paths roughly at right angles to each other, produce a resultant. The sum of all such resultants is called the *electrical axis* of the heart—the colored curve that runs diagonally across the heart in the diagram.

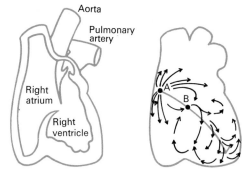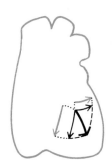

The diagram on the left is a reference for the schematized hearts shown next to it. The major conduction pathways through the core of the heart are shown in the center diagram. The heart's own built-in pacemaker, the sinu-atrial (SA) node (A), in the right atrium initiates a depolarization wave that travels through both atria. A single node in the wall between the right atrium and ventricle, the atrio-ventricular (AV) node (B), picks up this wave and relays it through a special conducting network that runs down the septum between the two ventricles and into the ventricular muscle. The diagram on the right shows how two waves traveling down diverging pathways (orange arrows) produce a resultant force in the direction of the thicker black arrow. The EKG measures the instant sum of all such resultants.

Two things can affect the direction of this axis: the patient's physique, and damage or disease. In people who are short and stout the stomach can push the heart up; in tall, lean people the heart can hang more vertically. If conduction in one of the ventricles is impaired, pathways through the other ventricle emit stronger signals and shift the axis in their direction. How do such changes alter the readings?

The photo opposite shows where the electrodes are attached to the patient for standard EKG sessions. The accompanying diagram shows the combinations of electrodes that drive the writers. In EKG parlance such combinations are called "leads"; they correspond to the "channels" of the EEG.

If we think of the arms as extensions of the shoulders and of the legs as extensions of the navel (electrically speaking, of course), we can use these points to construct a triangular graph that will be useful in interpreting EKG's. Such a graph (known as *Einthoven's triangle* for William Einthoven, the Dutchman who pioneered the EKG) is shown on page 40. Leads I, II, and III

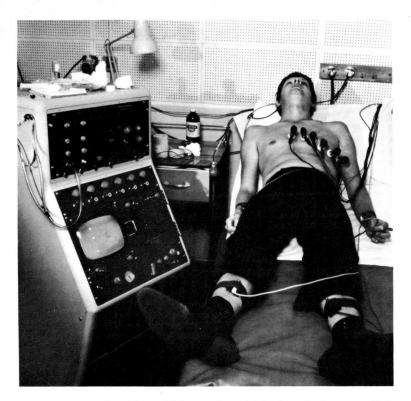

Above: a patient rigged for an EKG recording with leads on both arms and left leg and V leads on chest (lead on right leg is an earth). Switching devices in the recorder make appropriate combinations for recording on up to 10 channels (only 3 are in use here). Below: standard leads and combinations used for EKG recordings. I, II, and III are bipolar—that is, they give readings between two points of Einthoven's triangle (which is superimposed on the figure and illustrated overleaf). The other leads give voltage (or V) readings because the voltage they detect is related to a base voltage, which is derived from combinations of leads (signals from combined leads, being stronger, have to be attenuated by a resistance, which is usually 5000 ohms per lead).

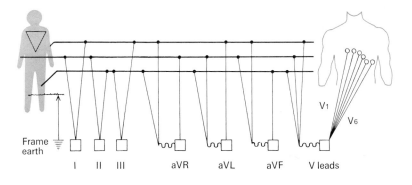

Frame earth

I II III aVR aVL aVF V leads

V₁
V₆

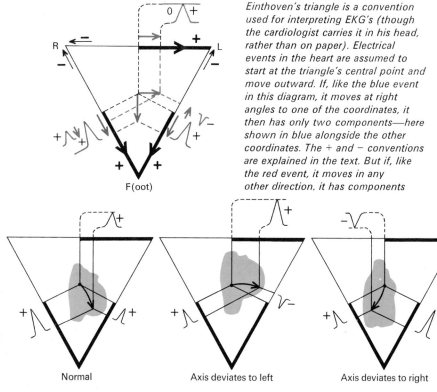

Einthoven's triangle is a convention used for interpreting EKG's (though the cardiologist carries it in his head, rather than on paper). Electrical events in the heart are assumed to start at the triangle's central point and move outward. If, like the blue event in this diagram, it moves at right angles to one of the coordinates, it then has only two components—here shown in blue alongside the other coordinates. The + and − conventions are explained in the text. But if, like the red event, it moves in any other direction, it has components

Normal   Axis deviates to left   Axis deviates to right

measure electrical movements parallel to the sides of this triangle. By convention we call movements in one direction along an axis *positive* (shown as heavy arrows in the diagram); in the opposite direction, of course, they are *negative*. Positive readings give an upward deflection of the writer; negative ones go downward; movements directly toward an axis have a zero component in either direction and do not affect the writer.

Now we can answer the question posed a few paragraphs back. The three other triangles in the diagram we have just looked at show that with a normal heart the traces from all three leads are positive (upward). The other conditions—which, remember, could be due either to a displaced heart or to a damaged one—give negative (downward) traces on one lead.

along each of the coordinates. The direction of the deflection depends on whether the component is + or −; its magnitude depends on the magnitude of the component. Opposite are shown such triangles for the three conditions described in the text.

Right: typical readings from V electrodes around heart (viewed from above). They show a general movement of electricity away from the upper right of the heart and toward the lower left.

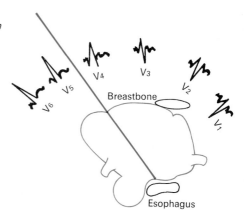

The aV leads incorporate a circuit to amplify the faint signals and are essentially devices for picking out one of the Einthoven components with reference to the other two. The V leads, which are placed on the skin just in front of the heart, detect movement toward or away from their electrodes relative to a plane that intersects the shoulders and hips. Typical traces from each lead are shown above; as you would expect, they show a general movement away from the upper right of the heart toward the bottom left. For special investigations it is also possible to put an electrode down the esophagus to a point only millimeters away from the left atrium (the only large region not accessible to the V leads). And to investigate the inside of the heart one can put electrode-containing catheters down veins or arteries (by techniques described in Chapter 4).

The interpretation of an EKG is much easier than that of an EEG, though it is still a matter for the specialist. We are, after all, looking at the record of just three events: (1) the wave of depolarization as it moves through the atria (refer back to the diagram on page 38)—known as the P wave; (2) the further passage of this depolarization wave through the AV node and across the ventricles—known as the QRS complex; (3) the repolarization of the ventricular muscle—known as the T wave. (The corresponding repolarization of the atria is something of a mystery, because it never shows on the EKG. Textbooks usually

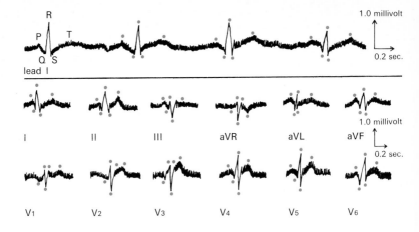

Normal EKG's display PQRST complex described in the text; these are identified at upper left and marked with colored points on all the other traces. The upper trace , from lead I, shows the normal timing; the lower traces show how the same complex appears in each of the 12 EKG leads.

say that it is "masked by the QRS complex"; but even in complete heart block, where the QRS occurs only occasionally, the wave that ought to signify atrial repolarization does not appear.) The traces shown above are normal readings of the PQRST complex for each lead. There are about 40 different conditions that affect these traces in one way or another. Changes occur in the timing, the amplitude, or the shape; examples are shown (together with explanations) opposite. Because the valves play no part in the electrical conduction of the heart, valve defects do not show in the EKG unless the heart has changed in some way to compensate for the defect, and even then we can only infer that the valve is defective. To confirm such an inference we rely on methods described in Chapter 4.

In general, electrical measurements are among the most satisfying of all the measurements we can make of the body's activity. Patients can be attached to the machines fairly quickly and the method involves no insult to, or interference with, the internal milieu. The results are instantaneous and, with skilled interpretation, can tell us a great deal about the state of the nerves or muscles. And, as we shall see later, the signals we get from the heart can be used for triggering quite a range of machines, from pacemakers to automatic monitoring devices.

P   T   P   P   T   P   P & T

Complete heart block. The P waves arise normally but, because the conducting network is blocked, their stimulus never reaches the ventricles, which contract autonomously at a very slow rate. Remedy: pacemaker.

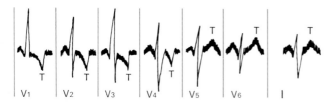

V₁   V₂   V₃   V₄   V₅   V₆   I

Hypertrophy (enlargement) of right ventricle shows in tall R waves and inverted T waves in V₁ to V₄ and distorted QRS in lead I. Remedy: unblock the outflow from the ventricle.

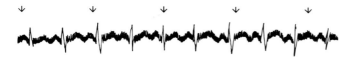

Pattern normal but rhythm fast (120/minute—arrows mark 1-second intervals). Common in emotion, fever, and certain kinds of poisoning.

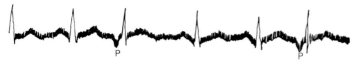

P   P

An irritable focus in the atrium can release trigger stimuli similar to those from the SA node—the natural pacemaker. Such stimuli often show as inverted P waves. Since the rest of the conducting network is normal, the QRST complex is unaffected. Remedy: drugs.

II   III   V₂   V₃   V₄   V₅

This patient had a coronary thrombosis that killed part of his heart. The damage shows in gross ST elevation in V₂ to V₅ and leads II and III— indicating that the damage lies to the front of the heart. Remedy: transplantation or surgery.

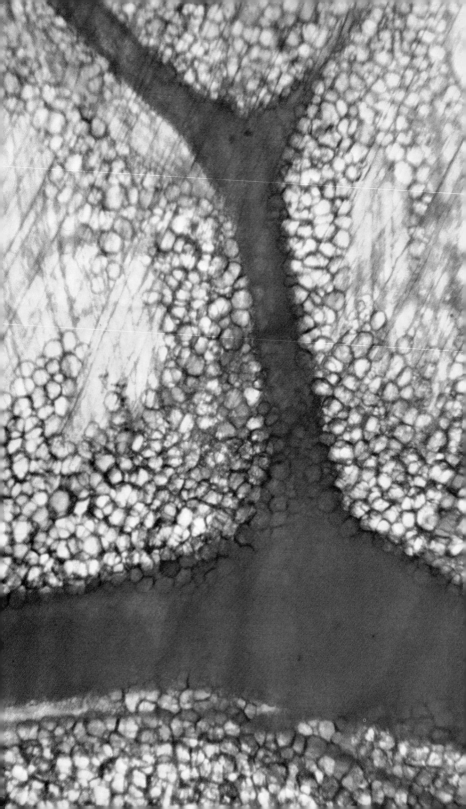

3 Chemical Samples

The body is such a finely balanced chemical system that even minor disorders can quickly upset the balance. So much so that the hundreds of thousands of chemical tests that doctors annually carry out on their patients are only rarely aimed at detecting traces of abnormal substances; their purpose, rather, is to find abnormal *quantities* of quite normal body chemicals—enzymes, proteins, metabolites, ions, dissolved gases, waste products, and so on. Excesses, deficits, or fluctuations in these are good guides to abnormal cellular activity, which is really what we are interested in.

The best place to find these chemicals is in the blood—the only tissue that directly or, through the lymph, indirectly bathes every other tissue in the body. Sometimes we do not need to tap the blood itself; we can, for instance, analyze exhaled breath, which has been in near contact with the blood, or perspiration, which is partly derived from blood, or urine, which derives wholly from blood. But these products are at several removes from activity within the cell; they contain fewer of the chemicals listed above;

Most of the machines described in this chapter are designed to detect in blood telltale imbalances of gases or body chemicals. Because the blood directly or indirectly bathes every tissue of the body (the tiny vessels shown here are magnified 100 times) it provides the doctor with an excellent means of monitoring cellular activity. Even so the interpretation of its contents must still be carried out with extreme care.

and those they do contain may exist in concentrations quite different from their concentrations in the blood. In short, their value as a guide to cell activity is more limited. The diagram on page 20 in Chapter 1 shows the critical balance our bodies maintain between proteins, electrolytes, and other solutes in the body fluids. No single center in the body regulates all these components. Some are controlled by the kidneys, which are themselves controlled by hormones; some by the liver; some by the lungs. The various organs of the gut also play a part. The balance can be upset by a large number of diseases or conditions, some of which attack the organs I have just listed, although others upset the metabolism in general. Major surgery (which the body cannot distinguish from any other injury) also upsets the balance. And though we are far from understanding the mechanisms involved, we do have a long clinical experience of their effects. In other words, by looking at the pattern of abnormality in blood constituents we get a good idea of the seat of trouble; and the degree of abnormality is usually an index of its severity.

Even so, blood is not an infallible guide. Remember, the cell wall actively strives to maintain normality within, against steep fluctuations without. So measurements of blood chemicals must always be interpreted with care—as many an intern is chagrined to discover. It is quite possible to find normal blood levels of, for example, potassium (K^+) in a potassium-starved patient, or to get transient abnormal readings in healthy people. In fact, the mention of normality brings us to the major problem of all chemical sampling.

What is "Normal"?

The readings opposite were obtained by pushing a fine tube, or *catheter*, down the median cubital vein (near the elbow) of a patient and, using low-dosage X rays, guiding it into the inferior vena cava. From its lower end upward this great vein drains blood from the lower limbs, the kidneys, and the liver (part of whose blood comes from the stomach veins). On reaching the heart it is joined by the superior vena cava, which drains the upper torso, arms, and head. Inside the heart these united streams are joined by a third stream, from the heart tissues themselves. At selected

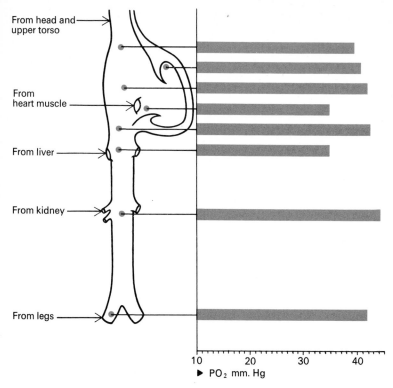

From head and upper torso

From heart muscle

From liver

From kidney

From legs

PO_2 mm. Hg

PO_2 of blood at various points in the inferior vena cava and right side of the heart. The liver and heart are big consumers of O_2; the kidneys are not—nor are the muscles when the body is at rest. The text poses a number of questions about variations of this kind.

points samples of venous blood were withdrawn and analyzed for oxygen content (PO_2) by methods that will be discussed later.

The term PO_2 needs a little explanation, because medical usage is, at first sight, confusing. PO_2 is read as "oxygen tension" (and, similarly, PCO_2 is "carbon dioxide tension"). But the P stands for "pressure." The usage is based on the law of partial pressures (Dalton's Law), which states that the pressure exerted by a gas in a mixture of gases is equal to the pressure the same quantity of that gas would exert in isolation. For instance, dry atmosphere exerts a pressure of 760 mm. Hg; oxygen, which makes up 20.96 per cent of the atmosphere, thus accounts for 20.96 per cent of $760=159.2$ mm. Hg. If we bubbled such air through a sample of blood, the air and blood would rapidly come into equilibrium such that the blood could take up no more oxygen. The blood

PO_2 would then be 159.2 mm. Hg. The air in the alveoli of the lungs contains 14.2 per cent of oxygen and water vapor equivalent to 45 mm. Hg. Because PO_2 is always expressed in terms of dry air, we must subtract the 45 from 760 to get the partial pressure of alveolar oxygen: 14.2 per cent of $(760-45)=101.53$ mm. Hg. The average PO_2 of venous blood is 40 mm. Hg, that of arterial blood is 100 mm. Hg; in other words the blood comes into almost perfect equilibrium with the alveolar air during its passage through the lungs—no mean achievement when the time it takes to do so can be as little as 0.3 second.

To return to the graph on page 47, the wide variation in PO_2 is marked enough, and no individual sample is average. What are we to make of these variations? How much can we attribute to the fact that the patient was old and fat? That he was a man? That he had eaten six hours ago? That he had been at rest for about two hours before the samples were withdrawn? Perhaps this patient feels certain symptoms when exercising, yet with this technique he must be kept at rest; so what validity do our readings have anyway?

To none of these important questions can we make a satisfactory answer. And the same kind of ignorance attends practically every other chemical measurement we can make. As a first step toward dispelling such ignorance we obviously need many more measurements on all kinds of patients and on healthy volunteers. That at least would enable us to assign probable weightings to such universal factors as age, weight, sex, diet, race, and so on. But a good deal of intuition would still be involved in interpreting the results with any given patient, for, although broad sample tests would reveal the variations to be expected among healthy individuals in general, we should have no way of knowing whether the patient normally occupied the high or middle or low end of the statistically average scale—still less of predicting his particular variations with diet, exercise, age, etc. To make matters more complicated, even this unknown individual norm could be masked by illness. Two solutions to the problem suggest themselves. The first, the pragmatic approach, would depend on vastly improved early-warning diagnosis. A patient with an incipient but serious condition could be extensively monitored for a wide variety of chemical parameters under a wide variety of circumstances—such tests to be repeated at regular intervals. Then when the condition became grave enough for surgery or other therapy we should have all the norms, the variations, and the tendencies for this particular patient to use as our reference lines. Moreover we should have objective standards for defining his return to normal. It would be heinously expensive. The second approach, more promising because more fundamental, would be to locate the genetic, cellular, or environmental basis of natural variation. Here we look to biochemists and molecular biologists, because, strictly, the subject lies outside the field of medicine. Neither of these approaches excludes the other, but if either is to work it will have to be backed by great improvements in existing machines.

Principles of Chemical Measurement

When we analyze, say, the blood in order to determine the quantities of its various constituents, the principles on which we base our analysis are remarkably simple. Most of them will be familiar to anybody who has completed an elementary science course. As in other kinds of measurement, there are two basic approaches: direct and indirect. For instance, we can directly measure the presence of a substance (call it x) in a mixture by shining light of a known wavelength (or a known band of wavelengths) on or through the mixture and measuring the changes between the incident and transmitted beams. Or we can measure the presence of x indirectly by allowing it to react with another chemical and then measuring some parameter of the reaction—heat evolved, color change, the amount by which the product of the reaction lowers the freezing point of water, and so on.

To continue our earlier example, it so happens that PO_2 can be measured by both kinds of technique: direct measurements can be made with a reflection photometer, indirect ones with a conductivity test (very similar to the pH test described on page 55).

The Reflection Photometer

Most oxygen in the bloodstream does not exist in simple solution but in loose combination with hemoglobin (Hb) forming oxyhemoglobin (HbO_2). All photometric methods for determining the PO₂ of the blood depend on the different light reflection characteristics of Hb and HbO₂. These are shown in the curves on this page. Note that at wavelength 6.1×10^{-7} meters (in the orange part of the spectrum) the difference between the two is at the maximum: HbO₂ absorbs much less orange light than Hb— hence its bright red appearance. But at wavelength 8×10^{-7} meters (in the infrared) Hb and HbO₂ absorb identical amounts of light. Here, then, is a basis for measurement: one wavelength at which two substances behave identically, another at which their difference is maximum.

Some calculations are necessary in the first place so that the machine readings can be interpreted in terms of the oxygen concentration of the blood. Of course, once the reflection photometer is set up (see diagram on page 52) the operator does not need to go through these calculations for each reading; that, after all, is the basic virtue of all machines—they do the donkeywork for us. He uses a cuvette filled with india ink to set the zero point on the galvanometer scale (this cancels out readings due to reflections from the glass of the cuvette); then he uses an identical cuvette filled with standard red dye, to give a standard galvanometer deflection. Having thus calibrated the instrument he can filter the light, first at 610 millimicrons, then at 800 millimicrons, and the deflections at these wavelengths can be interpreted directly as PO₂ readings.

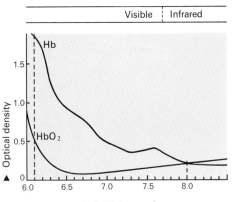

Optical densities of hemoglobin (Hb) and oxyhemoglobin (HbO₂) at various wavelengths are compared in this graph. Difference is maximum at 6.1×10^{-7} meters, zero at 8.0×10^{-7} meters.

A number of factors can distort the readings. Anemia, which results in a low total hemoglobin concentration, can push the readings into a nonlinear part of the scale. Hemolysis—destruction of the red cells, liberating hemoglobin into the plasma—gives very inaccurate readings. So does blood with clots in it. Vapor from formaldehyde (a common chemical in pathology departments) can contaminate syringes, catheters, etc., and add a spurious 10 per cent to the PO_2 reading. If the patient has recently been examined by injecting dyes into his bloodstream, the dyes may linger on and interfere with the PO_2 determination. These and other factors must be allowed for by the operator.

What does this detailed example teach us about chemical sampling in general? First, we see that even an apparently simple determination calls for complex and by no means instantaneous methods; thus, even in the swiftest determination we know how the patient was several minutes earlier, not how things are now. Second, because we are using only two parameters—optical density at 610 and 800 millimicrons—to measure a very complex phenomenon, the method is highly susceptible to error; thus the most important "machine" in the laboratory is the human operator, who alone can compensate for those errors.

The same points could be made about all the other chemical sampling machines in medicine. Let us look briefly at the principles on which each is based.

Spectrophotometry

Here again we use the properties of light as our basis of measurement—not just two filtered wavelengths but the entire visible spectrum and parts of the infrared and ultraviolet too. The customary unit for measuring spectral wavelengths—the angstrom unit ($A = 10^{-10}$ meters)—gives us a working range between about 2000 and 8000 A, the visible portion being from 3600 to 7700 A. Because even the fairly simple spectroscopes we use in our laboratories can distinguish down to 1 A, they constitute a powerful tool for sorting out the light from any substance heated to incandescence. Individual elements and simple ions, so heated, will emit light of characteristic wavelengths; the intensity of the light depends on the temperature and on the concentration

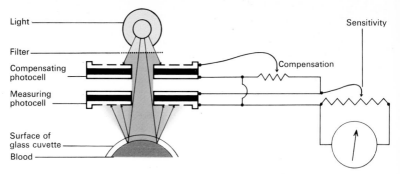

Basic design of reflection photometer is outlined. Two photocells are set back to back and wired in opposition to each other. To set up the instrument the light is shone into a cuvette filled with india ink. The signal from the compensating cell is adjusted, through the variable compensation resistance, to give a zero galvanometer deflection. This eliminates the effect of light reflected from the cuvette glass. The next reading is taken with a standard dye—the sensitivity resistance being adjusted to give a standard deflection. A blood-filled cuvette is then exposed to light filtered at 610 and 800 millimicrons and readings can be interpreted in terms of blood PO_2.

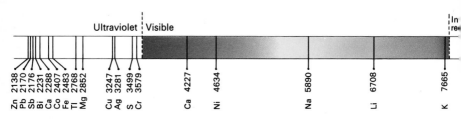

Absorption lines used for determining certain chemical elements in blood, urine, and other biomaterials. Calcium, sodium, and potassium, which are present in large quantities in tissue, can also be determined by their emission spectra at the same wavelengths, all of which are in the visible part of the spectrum.

of the element in question. If the element is fairly abundant (for sodium 2500 to 3500, and for potassium 80 to 200, parts per million) in the serum or urine or tissue extract, we can vaporize it and burn it in a flame of known temperature and so calculate its concentration directly from the intensity of one of its characteristic emission lines. The most familiar machine operating on this principle is the flame photometer, which is used for measuring sodium, potassium, and calcium.

If, however, the element is present only in traces (examples are chromium, magnesium, cobalt, and copper), its emission may be too faint to measure accurately. But, it so happens, gaseous

Right: a technician uses an atomic absorption spectrophotometer to determine magnesium in serum. The serum is sprayed into an air/acetylene flame and light of magnesium's line spectrum (produced by the hollow cathode tube at left) is beamed down the long axis of the flame. The magnesium absorbs some of this light, the absorption being proportional to the concentration of serum magnesium. Below: an absorption spectrophotometer for use with solutions. The cover has been removed to show the mirrors-and-prism system (diagramed below) that disperses the white source light into a continuous spectrum of which one wavelength is shone through the sample cell (see text).

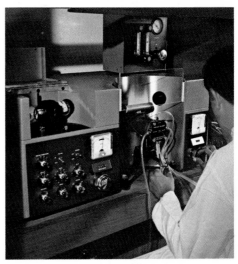

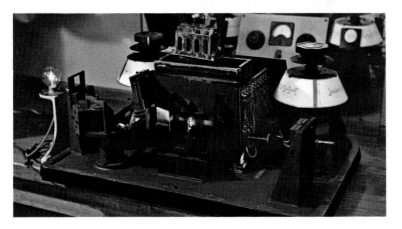

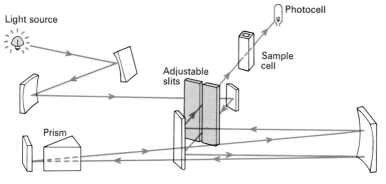

Light source

Photocell

Sample cell

Adjustable slits

Prism

elements will absorb light of the same frequency as they emit; if the incoming light is powerful, absorption is easy to measure. Thus, if we shine strong white light (in which the spectrum is continuous) from a high-temperature source through a lower-temperature flame containing certain elements, the light that emerges from the gas will be relatively deficient in certain wavelengths, and these will show as dark lines in the continuous spectrum. This indicates which elements are present; it does not reveal their concentrations. To do this we use the same principle but measure the absorption at one wavelength. The chart on page 52 shows the metal elements in which pathologists may be interested and the wavelengths used for detecting them. In practice the spectral line for the element under examination is produced by an especially designed cathode discharge tube (a different tube is used for each element) and this is beamed through a flame into which the sample solution is being sprayed. The absorption is measured by a photocell and can be interpreted directly in terms of the concentration of the sample solution. The machine shown at the top of page 53 operates on this principle.

On the same page is shown an absorption spectrophotometer used for measuring the concentration of substances in solution. Light of the required wavelength is produced by reflecting and dispersing the white source light (a tungsten filament lamp is used for most readings) through the mirrors-and-prism system shown in the diagram. Adjustable slits prevent all but the chosen wavelength from passing through the sample solution. A photocell connected to a meter records the degree of absorption, and comparison with standard solutions indicates sample concentration.

Measuring Acidity

A chemical variable that can be easily measured and that has great diagnostic value is the acidity or alkalinity of the blood or urine. These properties depend on the concentration of hydrogen ions (cH^+); a strong alkali has only 10^{-14} gm. H^+ per liter, a strong acid has about 1 gm. (10^0) of H^+ per liter. A scale that goes from 10^0 to 10^{-14} is not very convenient. By taking the log of the concentration we get a handier scale, from 0 to -14; but this means that all our quantities are negative, so, by convention, we reverse the sign to get a scale from 0 to 14. This scale is called *pH* and is equivalent to $-(\log cH^+)$. The neutral point is 7, the pH of pure water. Acids, rich in H^+, rate from 0 to 7 on the pH scale, and alkalis, poor in H^+, rate from 7 to 14.

The pH measurement is made with a "glass electrode." In essence this is a tubular membrane of a special glass (diameter 5.0 mm., wall thickness 0.4 mm.) that develops a voltage when the pH outside differs from the pH inside. Because glass is a non-conductor, the measurement is electrostatic. The blood volume needed for measurement is only 1.0 ml.—an important consideration when you are dealing with patients who cannot tolerate much blood loss, particularly very small children.

In a healthy person the blood pH never strays for long outside 7.37 to 7.45—a remarkably narrow range. Its narrowness is all the more remarkable when you consider that the end-products of metabolism are all acidic. Broadly speaking the metabolic process has two parts: an initial chain, known as the *lactate* chain, in which *glycogen* (animal starch) is converted to lactic acid; 80 per cent of this acid is reconverted to glycogen but the remaining part, together with proteins and fats, is put through a complex cycle of reactions, known as the *Krebs cycle*, whose end products are CO_2 and water, which combine to form carbonic acid as follows: $CO_2 + H_2O \rightleftharpoons H_2CO_3$.

Most of the steps in this process yield energy, but the end products, being acids, pose the body something of a problem. It cannot tolerate a wide variation in pH, yet here are these vital reactions, all pouring H^+ ions into the bloodstream. There are two lines of defense. The first is provided by substances called *buffers* that mop up H^+ ions. One of these, alkaline hemoglobin (KHb) in the red cell, tends to mop up H^+ ions and to fix them temporarily as acid hemoglobin (HHb). One product of this reaction is the bicarbonate ion HCO_3^-, which diffuses into the plasma and further depletes the H^+ ions by driving the reaction $H^+ + HCO_3^- \rightleftharpoons H_2CO_3$ forward. (In fact, this is only part of the story. The plasma itself contains proteins and phosphates that mop up H^+ ions in similar ways.)

The second line is formed by the lungs and kidneys. In the diagram on page 57 you will see that each reaction can go both

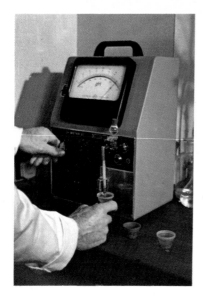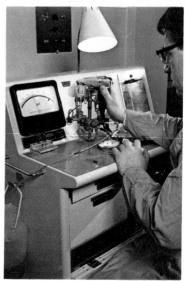

Above, left: calibrating a glass electrode pH meter by measuring the pH of a standard solution. Other standards of different pH are waiting for use.
Above, right: a technician uses an Astrup machine to determine pH and PCO_2 of blood. Of the 0.5-ml. blood sample taken from the patient, 0.1 ml. is sucked into a fine capillary and the pH determined by a glass electrode in the pistol-like attachment. The result is displayed on the meter at the left. Half the remainder of the sample is shaken with 4 per cent CO_2 in O_2 and the other half with 8 per cent CO_2 in O_2. The pH readings of these portions give actual PCO_2 and bicarbonate level in the blood. Advantages are small sample required and instantaneous results achieved.

ways—in other words, all the reagents are at or near equilibrium, and a change in any one of them can alter the equilibrium and tilt the reaction either forward or backward. At the lung there is a sharp change in the partial pressures of CO_2 and O_2—compared, that is, with the tissues that the blood has recently visited (see diagram on page 58). The blood ($PCO_2=46$) meets the lung surface ($PCO_2=40$) with the result that the equation $H^+ + HCO_3^- \rightleftharpoons H_2CO_3 \rightleftharpoons CO_2 + H_2O$ is again driven forward, reducing the H^+ ions in the blood.

The kidneys, quite simply, have the ability to pull H^+ ions out of the blood. Thus the urine, with a pH between 5 and 6, is always more acid than the blood—in health, anyway. The kidneys provide the coarse adjustment of pH; the lungs, which rely on the more delicate equilibrium-tilting reaction, perform the fine adjustment. But neither could cope on its own.

In many kinds of illness the lungs and kidneys can compensate for each others' failures. If a patient has poor lungs, the CO_2 will not be removed efficiently—leading to a fall in blood pH. The kidneys then step up their H^+ export and retain HCO_3^- above the normal level, which is 24 mEq/1. On the other hand, if a patient's kidneys are poor, or his circulation restricted, there will be a rise in his blood acidity (HX in the diagram on this page) and his lungs will vent more CO_2 to compensate.

A fall in pH is known as *acidosis*—a relative term, because the blood is always alkaline except in terminal illness (when failing lungs and kidneys cannot clear metabolic acids rapidly enough). Clearly, acidosis may be due to either a rise in PCO_2 because of faulty lungs or a fall in HCO_3^- because of faults in kidneys,

The most important elements of the interdependence of respiration, metabolism, and blood pH are shown below. Two buffer systems are shown in black: (1) red cells mop up H^+ ions; (2) strong acids (HX) produced by metabolism drive the equilibria in such a way that the weakly acidic bicarbonate (HCO_3^-) is produced in their stead. The kidneys (by maintaining an H^+ ion gradient between the blood and the urine) and the lungs (by maintaining a PCO_2 gradient between the tissues and the environment) also help the equilibria to tilt away from strong acid and toward weak acid. Three crucial and interdependent parameters of these equilibria are pH, bicarbonate concentration, and PCO_2—all of which can be measured in the plasma.

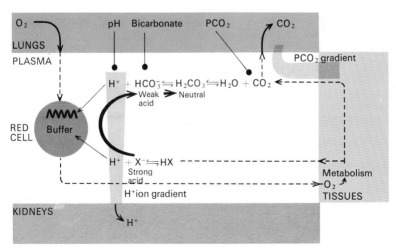

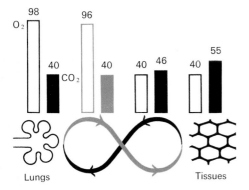

Partial pressures in millimeters of mercury of O_2 and CO_2 in lungs, oxygenated blood (orange), deoxygenated blood (black), and tissues.

circulation, blood pressure, or the metabolism. Conversely, *alkalosis* (a rise in pH above normal) may be due to a fall in PCO_2 through hysterical overbreathing (or over-ventilation if the patient is on a ventilating machine) or to a rise in HCO_3^- through some other organic failure. If the PCO_2 alone changes, we call it a *respiratory* acidosis or alkalosis; if the HCO_3^- alone changes, we call it a *metabolic* acidosis or alkalosis—the distinction is important in localizing the seat of the failure.

It is one of the triumphs of modern physiology that by measuring a single parameter—blood pH—we can tell to within fine limits not just whether a patient is suffering from a respiratory or metabolic acidosis or alkalosis, but how much this is compensated for by the lungs or kidneys. Look again at the diagram on page 57 and you will see that the three parameters, PCO_2, pH, and HCO_3^- concentration, not only straddle the reaction, not only are in equilibrium, *but are accessible in the plasma.* In other words, here is the one place where we don't have to go delving inside cells to know what's wrong. Know any two of these parameters and, because they are in equilibrium, you automatically know the third. The problem is that while pH can be measured in seconds, PCO_2 and HCO_3^- concentration call for more cumbersome methods. Here's how the problem poses itself clinically.

Suppose we take the standard chart on which these things are recorded (first graph on page 60). A healthy person will have readings of pH=7.4 and PCO_2=40 mm. Hg (point A on the graph). Now take a patient whose pH is also 7.4; is this patient normal or has he a compensated acidosis or alkalosis? If we knew either his PCO_2 or his HCO_3^- concentration, we could decide. But, as we saw, the problem is that we cannot measure either with such ease. The way around the problem is to abolish it. We divide the patient's blood sample into three. One part we measure for pH. One we shake in an atmosphere with a PCO_2 well above the normal level; the other we shake in an atmosphere with a PCO_2 well below the normal level (54 and 27 mm. Hg respectively). If we measure the pH of these samples, we can plot an upper and lower point on the graph and connect them with a line *on which the patient's actual pH must lie.* Reading across from this actual plot we can tell his actual PCO_2. The second graph on page 60 shows such plots for a healthy person.

Suppose our patient's samples show a pH of 7.38 and 7.56. The situation is now as shown in the third graph—that is, his "normal" pH of 7.4 (A′) gives a PCO_2 of 50, or 10 too high. If we artificially reduced his PCO_2 to the normal 40, he would suddenly have an excess of HCO_3^-, which until now had been compensating for the excess CO_2 in his blood. In other words he has a respiratory acidosis compensated by a metabolic alkalosis. Now take the contrary case: suppose his samples show a pH of 7.25 and 7.46. The fourth graph shows that his "normal" pH of 7.4 (A″) gives a PCO_2 of only 33, or 7 too low. If we artificially raised his PCO_2 to the normal 40, he would suddenly have a deficit of HCO_3^-. This is a metabolic acidosis compensated by a respiratory alkalosis.

Study of these third and fourth graphs enables us to add a third scale to the graph—the scale representing HCO_3^- concentration. This is done in the fifth graph, which combines all the readings so far taken. If we plot the HCO_3^- scale along the normal PCO_2 line—that is, at 40—we note that the line for the patient with metabolic alkalosis cuts this scale to the right of normal, while that for the patient with metabolic acidosis cuts the scale to the left. The sixth chart sums this up: the four lines radiating from the normal point define pure states of respiratory and metabolic acidosis and alkalosis. Usually, since these states are compensated, a patient's actual plot will lie between these lines; the graph shows how to interpret such plots, too.

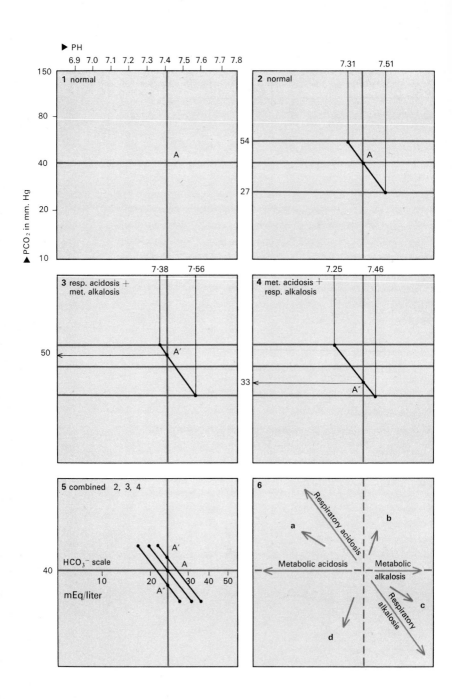

Automated Analyzers

The chart on page 63 shows the commonest blood constituents that pathologists can measure; it also shows the normal range in health, and some of the diseases or conditions associated with abnormal levels. The simplest methods for measuring these constituents are all indirect—that is, we allow the constituent to react with a specific reagent and then measure the product of the reaction. There are perhaps thousands of such reactions, allowing the pathologist a wide range of methods. In choosing among them he asks such questions as: Are the reagents expensive? Do they store well? Is the resulting optical density linear—that is, does the density increase in direct proportion to the original concentration of the constituent he wants to determine? Is the reaction fairly quick? Is the sensitivity of the right order (he wants low sensitivity if the samples are going to have a wide range of concentrations, high sensitivity if the samples will fall within a narrow range)? And, increasingly, is the process capable of automation?

The six pH/PCO₂ charts shown opposite are discussed at length in the text. Directions a, b, c, and d represent combinations of the two nearest conditions. Below: a technician records results from an Astrup machine on a PCO₂/bicarbonate/pH graph to detect acidosis or alkalosis.

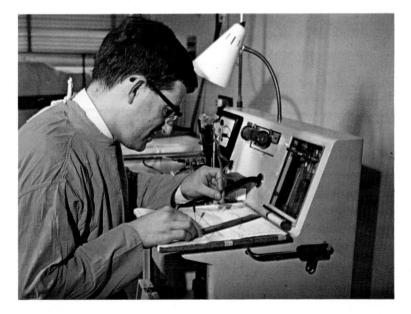

As hospitals grow in size and as doctors make greater demands on their pathology departments, this question of automation grows in importance. The standard equipment for automated analysis is the Technicon AutoAnalyzer (shown on page 64), which operates at 40 to 60 analyses an hour. Basically it consists of a long fine tube through which are drawn samples of blood serum, urine, etc., separated by quantities of neutral solution—in most cases distilled water. The samples and stretches of water between them are themselves separated by air bubbles. This provides extra protection against contamination between samples, and the air bubbles have a useful scouring effect on the walls of the tubing. The heart of the machine is the proportioning pump that by way of a manifold introduces the air bubbles into the sample and reagent streams and advances precise quantities of all solutions and diluents into the system (see the diagram on page 64). Before some chemicals can be estimated, protein molecules, which would interfere with the reaction, must be removed. This is done by passing the sample through a dialyzer—a porous cellulose membrane that holds back the proteins but allows smaller molecules to pass through into the reagent stream (a miniature artificial kidney, in effect).

Reactions are chosen that produce a noticeable color change and these are monitored in a colorimeter, which is in effect an optical densitometer tuned to a particular color. The air bubbles are removed from the sample just before it passes into the colorimeter flowcell. Some reactions need warmth to develop their color and so a heating bath is incorporated in the line. Standard laboratory solutions of known concentration are passed through first and at regular intervals (usually after every tenth sample) to calibrate the recording apparatus. Readings from the colorimeter are displayed as peaks on a moving graph paper and once a standard curve has been prepared (using the standard solution readings) the peaks from the sample can be interpreted in terms of concentration.

This system, as it is used in most large hospitals, suffers from a number of inherent disadvantages. First, it can safely determine only one chemical at a time; the manifold, tubes, and reagents are changed for each different determination. If a number of tests are

Blood Constituents	Normal Range	Diseases due to *high* and low concentrations
Albumen	4-5·5g/100ml	*nephrotic syndrome,* severe malnutrition
Aspartate transferase	4-17 IU/1	*cardiac infarct*
Bilirubin	0·1-1mg/100ml	*jaundice*
Total protein	6-8g/100ml	*myeloma,* nephrotic syndrome
Lactic dehydrogenase	70-300 IU/1	*myelosclerosis, cardiac infarct*
Serum cholesterol	150-300mg/100ml	*myxedema,* thyrotoxicosis
Alkaline phosphatase	3-13 KA units	*Paget's disease, obstructive jaundice*
Bicarbonate	24-28mEq/1	diabetic ketosis, uremia
Blood glucose (fasting)	70-100mg/100ml	insulinoma, diabetes mellitus
Serum inorganic phosphate	3-4·5mg/100ml	*uremia,* osteomalacia
Serum urea	20-40mg/100ml	*renal disease,* severe acute hepatitis
Uric acid	2-7mg/100ml	*gout*
Calcium	9·5-10·5mg/100ml	*hyperparathyroidism,* osteomalacia
Chloride	90-110mEq/1	*dehydration,* pyloric stenosis
Potassium	3·5-5·5mEq/1	*Addison's disease,* Conn's syndrome
Serum iron	60-180mg/100ml	*hemochromatosis,* iron deficiency anemia
Sodium	133-145mEq/1	*Conn's syndrome,* Addison's disease

Blood constituents commonly determined by indirect methods—by either colorimetry or spectrophotometry. The center column shows the normal range for each constituent. The column on the right lists diseases or conditions associated with abnormally high or low concentrations of the constituent.

performed on the same sample as it passes along, each test may alter the sample in some way and introduce inaccuracy in the results of later tests. Second, the reading of the patient data (number, ward, and hospital) must usually be handled by the operator. And third, synchronization of patient data and analysis data at the readout must be controlled by means of an electronic pulse. The last two features are possible sources of error. Technicon have, in fact, developed a machine operating on the same general principles that can carry out up to 12 determinations simultaneously and that has a more positive patient and analysis readout identification system.

During 1969 a new machine, the Vickers Multichannel 300, designed to overcome the disadvantages in the standard system described above, began to appear in hospitals. As you can see in the photographs on page 65, it is essentially a modular system. Vials containing blood are marked with patient identification data

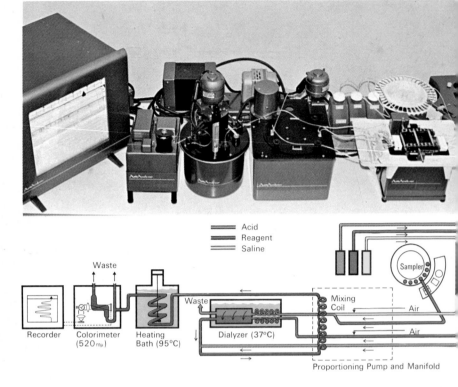

The top photograph shows how standard AutoAnalyzer equipment is arranged for determination of most blood constituents. The separate items are identified in the diagram, which is a simplified flow chart for the determination of urea in serum. The proportioning pump, shown in action lower left, consists of two parallel roller chains carrying several steel rollers that run against a spring-loaded platen. The resilient plastic pump tubes between the rollers and the platen are squeezed so that precise quantities of fluids or air are advanced into the system. At right below, a technician is using standard solution peaks to prepare a standard curve, which is then used to interpret sample peaks in terms of concentration.

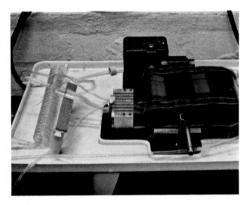

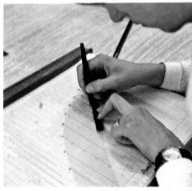

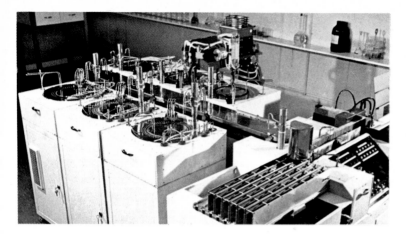

Above: the prototype of the Vickers Multichannel 300 automated biochemical analyzer described in the text. The reaction units are supplied with diluted plasma from the central conveyor belt. The flame photometer is at top center. The reaction rotor shown below contains 120 reaction cavities (the outer ring is used for blank determinations). Reagent dispenser probes have red magnetic bases, the secondary transfer diluter is at top left, and below it are the cavity laundry and colorimeter probes. At the bottom of the page, vials are shown moving toward the readout. Below the primary transfer diluter at extreme left, vials await perforation and sampling. Two rejected (and therefore unperforated) vials can be seen at right of center. The sample vial, shown life-size at below right, clearly demonstrates how light shone edgewise into it is reflected from the depressed sections of the label.

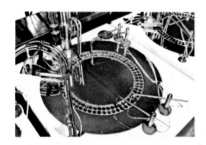

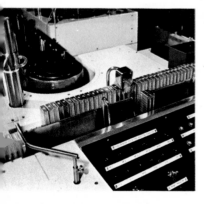

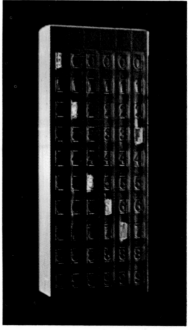

by depressing perforated numbered sections arranged in columns on the label. A similar label on the other face of the vial can be used to record hospital data (see the photograph on page 65). At the readout, light shone edgewise into the vial is reflected by the depressed sections onto photocells and the patient and hospital numbers are converted into electrical impulses.

The marked vials are first centrifuged, pushing the blood cells to the bottom and leaving the clear plasma above for analysis. Just before each vial moves from the magazine into the main part of the machine it passes through a plasma monitor, which checks that the vial has been filled to the correct level, that the blood cells and plasma are separated, and that the sample is not hemolyzed or otherwise unsuitable for analysis. Rejected vials are steered into a separate section and can be removed for examination. Vials that pass the test are perforated, and move forward; a suction tube withdraws a fixed amount of plasma and transfers it (together with some diluent) into a sample container. This container and others like it travel along a continuous belt around the "spine" of the machine. Intermittently the belt stops and a suction tube at each of the 12 similar sampling units withdraws and dilutes a part of the sample and dispenses the mixture into a reaction cavity. The top of each reaction unit consists of a rotor with one or two rings of reaction cavities, into which the samples and various reagents are dispensed. At the end of the reaction period (the rotor moves in stages as different cavities are used) a probe withdraws the reaction mixture into the flowcell of a colorimeter in the base of the unit. Each rotor can be maintained at a constant temperature independently of the others.

Meanwhile the vials have passed onto a caterpillar track that carries them toward the readout. The whole system is arranged so that, when a vial passes through the readout, analytical data from each reaction unit are being presented. Because linkage is mechanical, there is no possibility of getting Mr. A's results alongside Mrs. B's identity number. Electrical impulses from the reaction units and the vial indentification system are fed directly to the computer for presentation of analytical results. This, as well as storing, processing, and printing out results, also keeps an eye on all the machine's functions—giving advance warning of developing faults and automatically correcting drift in the colorimeter and flame photometer.

The machine takes a new sample every 12 seconds and produces results at the same rate. Each sample takes up to 10 minutes to analyze for 14 separate blood constituents (the flame photometer, which measures emission as the sample burns, determines Na^+, K^+, and Ca^{++} simultaneously). Because at any given moment some 50 samples are undergoing analysis, the machine works through a batch at the rate of 300 per hour. This is much faster than earlier machines could work, so that doctors and patients who formerly had to wait all day can now get results within the hour.

The benefits of batch processing in modular units are obvious. A hospital can start small with, say, six or eight reaction units, and then expand without having to scrap earlier purchases. If a unit fails, the technician can unplug it and replace it with a spare within minutes and repair it off line. New test methods can be introduced by altering or replacing any one of the units.

Automation does, however, bring one disadvantage that hospital organizers have been slow to appreciate. If there is anything duller than doing, say, 36 identical determinations of one blood constituent, it is the "job" of watching a machine do it all for you. Such machines ought to release technicians from routine work and allow them to get on with more interesting and important work. They are not always used in this way. The pathology labs of many small, unautomated hospitals have their quota of happy escapees from the larger, automated outfits. The problem is one of hospital organization—it cannot be laid at the door of the machine manufacturers. Nor is it unique to hospitals; wherever skilled men are needed to take over in case some automated control fails, there is dissatisfaction—which is less a matter of boredom than of a sense of inadequacy. As yet the problem is small—which is only another way of saying that hospital automation is in its infancy. It is going to grow into a giant. Many of the proposed solutions, which involve "deautomating" certain functions so that people feel needed, are retrogressive. We shall have to do better than that, for this problem is obviously not going to vanish of its own accord.

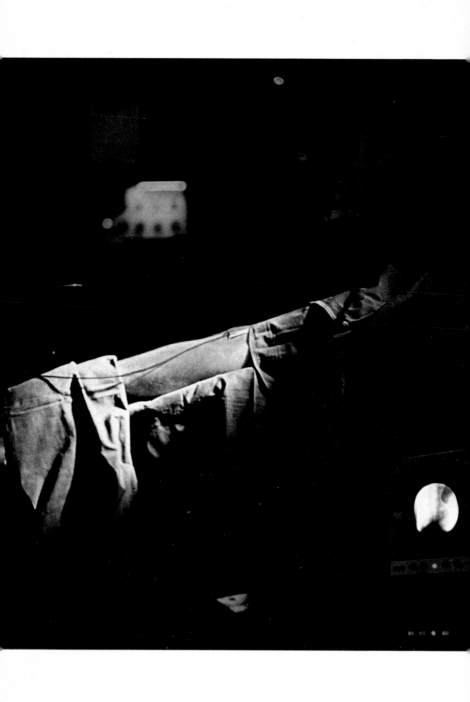

4   Vital Functions

Living systems have two distinctive features: they reproduce themselves and they resist invasion. From one point of view these activities are the "outputs" of life. The inputs are eating, drinking, and breathing. So far we have mainly looked at the outputs. The electrical and biochemical events whose measurement we have discussed are so rapid and so impalpable that our ordinary senses do not respond to them. Instead we have been forced to develop complicated machines and indirect methods to cope with them. Few of them measure—even approximately—what is happening inside the cells; to work with such machines is to enter a world where inference is not a mere technique, but a way of life.

In this chapter we look mainly at the inputs. At once we are in the familiar Newtonian world of pushes and pulls, where events have straightforward mechanical causes. Here we measure in graspable units like centimeters and liters rather than in cerebral microns and milliequivalents; and the things we measure we can also touch or see. The machines are correspondingly down-to-earth: tubes, springs, bellows, pulleys, and microphones are their functioning parts.

Heart-valve or septal defects do, in some cases, affect EKG readings but they can be detected more effectively during phonocardiograph and catheterization sessions. (The value and problems of these techniques are discussed in this chapter.) The patient shown opposite is undergoing cardiac catheterization in a darkened room. This allows the surgeon to monitor the catheter's position on a fluoroscope screen, visible at bottom right.

For some obscure reason such homely touches have devalued this branch of medicine in the public mind. The star doctor of the tiny screen will wade ankle-deep through EKG charts and discuss serum cholesterol at almost any length; but the nearest he gets to the food-and-air part of medicine is the diet sheet and the stethoscope. In his world, tests of cardiac and pulmonary function are strictly for the technicians. The situation has its comic side, for in real medicine the boot of prestige is usually on the other foot. This point is worth clearing up because these melodramas can color our attitudes more than we may admit. In fact there is no serious distinction between the varieties of medicine. All have at their root the sick or disordered cell; they are different aspects of the same ancient science of healing.

Nevertheless, the distinctions I have already drawn happen to be convenient—and useful—as long as you remember that they are no more than handy ways of dividing this complex science to make its contents manageable. Starting, then, with the three inputs of water, food, and air, we are led straight to the organs that process them: gut, liver, kidneys, lungs, and circulation. These stand, as it were, at the divide between the environment and all the other organs and tissues of the body. If any one of them fails to perform, the results reverberate throughout the system. Small wonder, then, that some of the most important diagnoses in medicine center around these particular organs. Let us look at them in turn.

The Gut, the Liver, the Kidneys

I put these under one heading because, with the circulation, they handle the chemical inputs, food and water. (The circulation, of course, is the common denominator in that it also handles the gases; it is better considered separately.) The gut turns the food into small, soluble molecules that pass readily into the bloodstream. The process begins in the stomach, which breaks up large food particles and pours secretions out to dissolve most of them; it continues in the duodenum and small intestine, which extract the now soluble food molecules; and it is completed in the large intestine, which bulks up the waste by extracting from it enough water and electrolytes to meet the body's needs. The vein from the small intestine—the portal vein—goes directly to the liver.

The liver, the largest organ in the body, is unique in its huge variety of functions. It is the great chemical clearing-house of the system. It modifies, synthesizes, or destroys the foodstuffs from the gut and chemicals from other organs and tissues. It stores the products and releases them as necessary. It recognizes and inactivates external and internal poisons. If the bone marrow fails to produce enough red cells, the liver begins to make them—a function it performs in the fetus before the bone is completely formed. It removes foreign matter, bacteria, and dead or degenerate red cells, turning them into bile, which, in its turn, is essential to normal digestion. It also plays a vital part in the manufacture of antibodies.

The kidneys excrete the end-products of all this activity—both from the liver and from the tissues that depend upon it. The kidney's structure and function are discussed in detail in *Spare-Part Surgery*, page 50. From our present point of view I would stress its regulatory function, by which it excretes a large number of chemicals—some wanted, some waste—and then actively selects and transports back the wanted products (electrolytes, water, sugars, buffers, etc.) into the bloodstream. The filtering-out occurs early in the capillary network, where the blood pressure is still high (40 mm. Hg); the selecting back occurs farther down the network, where the pressure is much lower (12 mm.Hg). This pressure difference is important to the proper functioning of the kidney, as we shall see.

Because most of the activity in the gut, liver, and kidneys is chemical, the machines used for testing their functions are, essentially, those we looked at in the previous chapter. For instance, all the chemicals listed on page 63 figure in tests of liver function; and many are important in tests of kidney and gut activity too. Tests made on blood, stomach juices, urine, and feces cannot, however, locate the actual site of a disorder; they can only tell us that a given organ is or is not performing well.

If the trouble is in the stomach or the lower parts of the ureters (the tubes running from the kidneys to the bladder) we can actually locate it without opening up the patient. The device we use is an endoscope—illustrated on pages 72 and 73 in two of its many forms: the bronchoscope and the gastroscope. Modern medical endoscopes are modifications of industrial endoscopes designed, in the first place, for inspecting jet engines without dismantling them. Some are based on the principles of fiber optics—bundles of fine (0.25-mm.) glass rods that, however bent or twisted, transmit light along their length. In most such endoscopes there are two fiber-optic systems, one for carrying the field illumination into the patient, the other for carrying a picture out again.

The bronchoscope is an observer's tool. The operating cystoscope is a more complex device that allows us to perform certain internal operations without opening the patient's skin: we can, for instance, work one up the urethra into the bladder and remove tumors with a very-high-frequency (35,000-Hz.) electrical current, or in testing kidney function we can use it to pass a catheter into each ureter to analyze the products of each kidney separately.

The small intestine and the kidney itself lie beyond the reach of any endoscope. To "see" faults within them we still rely in the

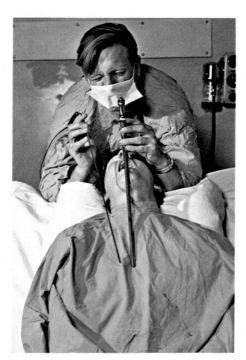

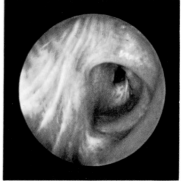

Left: a patient in position for bronchoscopy. The bronchoscope is held in front but in true alignment. A torch in the handle shines light down a groove in one side of the hollow metal tube, leaving a direct unobstructed view as shown below. The surgeon uses the sucker in his right hand to clear secretions from the bronchi. Only the bronchi and throat are anesthetized.

first place on X rays. The patient, starved for six hours to clear his gut, eats a "meal" of emulsified barium sulfate, which is radio-opaque. At various times over the following three to six hours the progress of this meal is photographed on X-ray film. The large intestine can also be examined by injecting two to three pints of barium through the anus with an enema. We can get similar records for the kidney by injecting radio-opaque iodoxyl or diodone intravenously and seeing how and where it is excreted. The photos on the next page show the kind of defect these techniques can reveal in the intestine and the kidney.

A variation of this technique is to give the patient a drink or injection containing a radioactive isotope of some nontoxic chemical—preferably one in which the turnover is quick, so that the radioactivity is soon dissipated. For kidney tests we use iodine-131-labeled hippuran, a saccharide. Some minutes later, by when the kidney should be excreting the labeled hippuran, we move a scintillation counter back and forth over the loin; where the activity is too weak or too strong the kidney is either failing or overactive.

Right: the gastrocamera in use here consists of a fiberscope with a camera, complete with film and flash lamp, located in the tip. The surgeon exposes and advances the film by remote control. He can also view through the camera lens by means of a prism and the glass fiber bundle. A viewing lamp is located next to the flash lamp. Shown below is the surgeon's-eye view of the stomach.

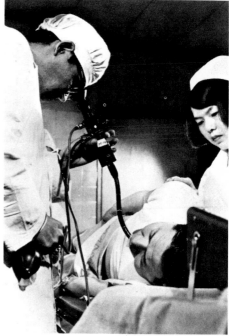

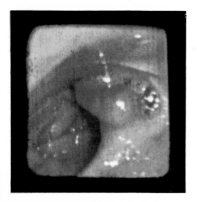

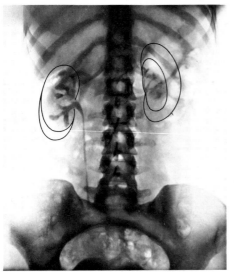

Kidney X ray (left), produced by methods outlined in the text, reveals that the patient's left kidney (inner outline) is less than $\frac{1}{4}$ its normal volume (other outline); the right kidney has also lost some substance from its lower border. Such X rays are our only means of determining the exact degree of loss. Unlike other X-ray photographs in this chapter, the one below is shown in negative form for the sake of clarity. The patient's bowel was enema-injected with radio-opaque barium, which was then evacuated. The bowel was then partly filled with air, which reveals where the barium has formed pools. The convoluted bowel in the lower part of the picture is normal; the smoothed bowel at the top is diseased.

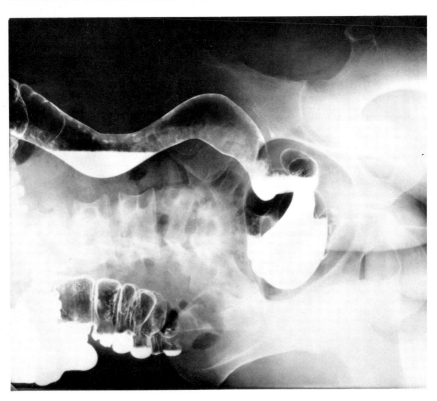

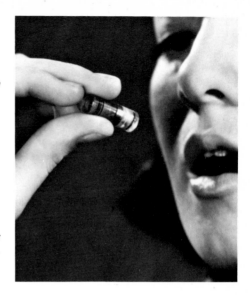

The pill this girl is swallowing contains a very-low-power radio transmitter whose broadcast wavelength (in the 400-500-kHz. range) varies with the pressure on the pill. A receiver placed close to her stomach will thus reveal local pressures as it travels through the bowel. Previously such measurements had to be made by inserting tubes, which was unpleasant for the patient and interfered with normal function. The pill responds to pressure up to 210 mm. Hg. Similar pills can check temperature (34–41°C) and pH (natural range). Such devices will greatly help us to define "normal," because they hardly interfere with any system into which they are introduced.

Finally we can learn something about the small and large intestine from radio pills. It is possible to monitor chemical activity in the gut by sucking out samples from a tube, which can occasionally be connected to a manometer to give pressure readings. However, the readings obtained from a bowel insulted in this way will rarely bear any real relationship to its normal behavior. To get more representative readings we use radio pills. The one shown on this page contains a battery-powered radio transmitter and is sensitive to pressure. Other transducers can be used for recording pH and temperature. Unfortunately this device is large enough to affect the bowel movements and secretions. Nevertheless the results obtained from its transmissions (monitored by a three-directional receiver system worn as a belt around the body) correspond very closely with studies made by serial X rays of radio-opaque media. Much smaller pills have been made without a battery but containing a tuned radio circuit. This modifies and retransmits radio frequency waves in a variable way dependent on pressure, temperature, or pH. These pills are complicated to use and so far have given no materially different results from the more conventional types.

The Heart-Lung

As functioning units the lung and heart are more easily considered as a single complex organ; but, because they contain, as it were, two compartments—one for blood, one for air—the tests we make are better discussed separately.

The air we breathe in goes down a tree-like arrangement of passages that end in minute sacs called *alveoli* (shown opposite). As it passes down it is humidified, warmed, and scoured of dust and small aerosol particles (i.e. particles small enough to be held permanently in suspension). At the alveolar surface, which is a mesh of fine blood capillaries, it exchanges some of its oxygen for some of the blood's CO_2. In the smaller branches most of the airflow is streamlined, so that the front of the incoming air presents an ever-lengthening wedge-shaped profile (see diagrams opposite). The center of this wedge actually penetrates to the alveolus and scours its inside with fresh air; convection currents between cooler incoming and warmer outgoing air also help to mix the gases.

The mechanics of the system are ingenious. The lungs lie in so-called pleural cavities within the chest ("so-called" because in health the cavity is potential rather than actual: the membrane around the lung is everywhere in contact with the lining of the "cavity"—only in disease do the cavities fill with fluid or air and so show on X-ray plates). Thus the lungs form elastic sacs within the airtight barrel of the chest. That barrel is bounded by the ribs and the diaphragm; any movement of these two boundaries will tend to alter the volume of the lungs (except with certain conditions in which the diaphragm movement counteracts the rib movement). The pair of X-ray plates on page 78 shows these movements and their effects on the lungs.

When the muscles that have expanded the chest barrel relax, the lungs contract again; they do so partly because of their own elasticity and partly because of the surface tension in the alveolar fluid, which tends always to collapse the alveolus. Because of this the pressure within the potential pleural cavity is always between 2.5 and 6 mm. below atmospheric. During normal relaxed breathing the diaphragm movement accounts for about 60 per cent of the volume increase with each inhalation. The remaining 40 per cent is achieved by rib movements, though the mechanism differs with sex and age. Women expand the top of the rib cage more than men; but with advancing years there is a

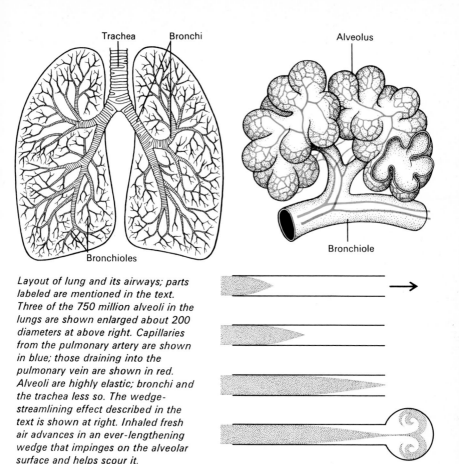

Trachea · Bronchi · Alveolus · Bronchiole · Bronchioles

Layout of lung and its airways; parts labeled are mentioned in the text. Three of the 750 million alveoli in the lungs are shown enlarged about 200 diameters at above right. Capillaries from the pulmonary artery are shown in blue; those draining into the pulmonary vein are shown in red. Alveoli are highly elastic; bronchi and the trachea less so. The wedge-streamlining effect described in the text is shown at right. Inhaled fresh air advances in an ever-lengthening wedge that impinges on the alveolar surface and helps scour it.

general tendency for the top of the rib cage to stiffen and breathing is increasingly transferred to the lower, more mobile ribs and diaphragm.

The heart, which is surrounded by the lung on both sides, pumps 80 ml. of blood into the lung capillaries with each beat—amounting to about 5 l/min. when relaxed. The capillary network, though fine, has so many branches that it offers remarkably little resistance to the blood. In fact the blood that enters the lung from the right ventricle is already returning to the left atrium by the time the right ventricle delivers its next 80 ml. to the lungs. In other words, at any given moment the lungs contain only 80 ml. or so of blood. This volume is spread out over the 55 m² of respiratory surface in 750 million alveoli and terminal bronchioles. This explains how the gas exchange between blood and

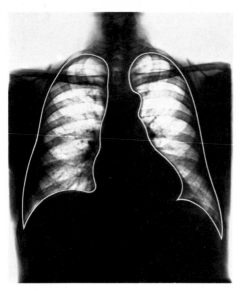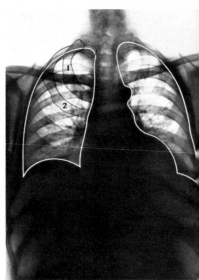

Changes in rib cage, diaphragm, and lung volume during normal breathing are shown in this pair of X rays. They are of the same subject and are taken within moments of each other.

alveolar air is achieved in less than 0.3 sec.

Because the lung-capillary resistance is low the blood pressure must be kept correspondingly small—15 mm. Hg compared with 80 mm. Hg in the systemic arteries. Even during hard exertion, when the blood throughput rises fourfold to 20 l/min, the pressure stays down around 20 mm. Hg. When the pulmonary blood pressure rises above these values, as it does in certain lung or heart conditions, it begins to force serum out of the capillary wall and into the alveolar space—a state known as *pulmonary edema.*

This very sketchy outline of the heart-lung complex, though far from complete, provides a basis for understanding the tests we make of lungs and heart function. By way of introduction to those tests let us look at possible failures in the system. They fall into three groups: inadequate air flow; inadequate gas exchange; and inadequate blood flow. These failures may occur singly or in any combination. Most of the following list of causes appear in the diagram on page 80.

Inadequate air flow occurs when the air passages are physically blocked with solid particles (dust, smoke, etc.) or mucus; when the air passages contract in a spasm under the influence of a brisk immune reaction or allergic reactions (such as asthma); when the passages and alveoli lose some of their elasticity so that they are unable to expand fully or contract naturally; or when the joints and muscles of the rib cage or diaphragm lose their mobility or strength.

Inadequate gas exchange occurs when the alveoli begin to break down and join together to form enlarged sacs (a condition known as *emphysema*); when the alveolar walls become diseased and thicken; when the alveoli fill with fluid—as in pulmonary edema; with anemia; with respiratory acidosis; or when the blood flow is inadequate.

Inadequate blood flow occurs when the general circulatory pressure falls to 50 per cent of normal (due to loss of blood or to abnormal dilation of the blood vessels); when the pulmonary valve is narrow (so allowing too little blood to leave the right ventricle) or leaks; when the pulmonary artery or veins are too narrow; when the capillary bed in the lung is affected by some lung disease; or when the mitral valve either is too narrow or leaks. Narrowness (called *stenosis*) and leaking often go together.

Some of these conditions will affect the total quantity of air we can get into our lungs; others will affect the distribution of that air; others will affect the rate at which we breathe in and out; and yet others will show mostly in the alterations they cause to blood pressure and chemistry. In short, we can test the air part of the system for some conditions, the blood part for others.

Respiratory Tests

If we connect a healthy person to a recording spirometer—the apparatus shown in the diagram on page 81—and ask him to breathe normally, the writer will trace out the kind of curve shown in the yellow section of the graph. When we ask him to breathe in as deeply as possible and out again to a normal level, the curve rises across the orange portion of the graph. When we ask him to force every last gasp from his lungs, the curve falls into the green part. These three regions define the vital capacity— that is, the volume of lung available for pumping gas to and from the atmosphere. The normal range is the *tidal* volume; the extra inhalation is the *complemental* volume; and the extra exhalation is the *reserve* volume. But even when the last gasp is out there is

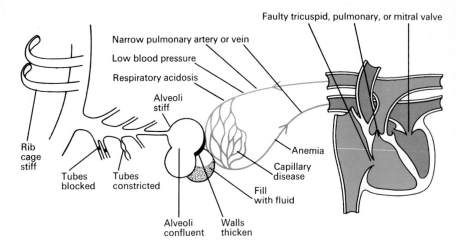

Faulty tricuspid, pulmonary, or mitral valve

Narrow pulmonary artery or vein

Low blood pressure

Respiratory acidosis

Alveoli stiff

Rib cage stiff

Tubes blocked

Tubes constricted

Anemia

Capillary disease

Fill with fluid

Alveoli confluent

Walls thicken

Some sites of possible failure in the heart-lung complex are reviewed in this schematic drawing; all are listed in the text.

still plenty of air (about 1500 ml.) in the lung; about 160 ml. of this is in the air passages, the remainder in the alveoli—together they form the *residual* volume, which has to be calculated because it cannot be directly measured.

The 160-ml. volume of the air passages is called the *anatomical dead space*—"dead" because there is no gas exchange across the thick walls of the trachea, bronchi, and bronchioles. The air in this space is always the next in line, as it were, for exhaling; after tidal breathing, the anatomical-dead-space air comes out before the reserve air—hence its shifting position on the graph (black rectangle). This volume becomes significant when a patient's breathing grows shallow. Normal tidal breathing involves the exchange of about 500 ml. of air per cycle, of which, by deducting 160 ml., we can assume 340 ml. to penetrate to the alveoli. Actually the figure is slightly higher because of the wedge-streamlining effect described earlier (page 76). If the breathing fell drastically, to below 160 ml. per cycle, even this effect would not be sufficient to get fresh air into the alveoli each time. Unless the rate increased or the patient were put on pure oxygen, he would very soon die.

The chart produced by the spirometer allows us to determine the degree of lung incapacity. Most lung conditions increase the residual volume (i.e. the volume of air that cannot be cycled in and out) two- or threefold. The charts on page 85 show typical patterns for spasmodic conditions such as asthma, and steady conditions such as emphysema (alveolar enlargement) and edema (waterlogging). They show that in asthma and emphysema the lungs are working at the top end of their capacity; the patient's chest feels very tight and he has to fight for each breath. With emphysema the tidal range is normal, but with the slightest exertion, the patient breathes to the full range of his vital capacity—which is much reduced. With asthma the bronchioles contract so much during breathing out that each cycle takes much longer. To compensate, the patient is forced to breathe more deeply, so even without exertion he breathes to the full range of his vital capacity—which, again, is very much less than normal. If he is given drugs to relax his bronchioles, his pattern returns to near normal.

With edema the lung tissues often grow less elastic, so their total capacity is reduced. Much of the residual volume is filled with fluid. The effect, as the graph shows, is to squash the normal

Principle of the spirometer is illustrated below. It consists of a counterweighted gasholder linked to a moving pen in such a way that respirations are recorded on a chart as waves whose height reflects the volume of air breathed in or out. Studies of the breathing of healthy people enable us to single out five zones, shown in black and color on the chart below; they range from maximum inhalation (orange) to maximum exhalation (green). The percentages given are in terms of total lung air capacity. The chart reads from right to left.

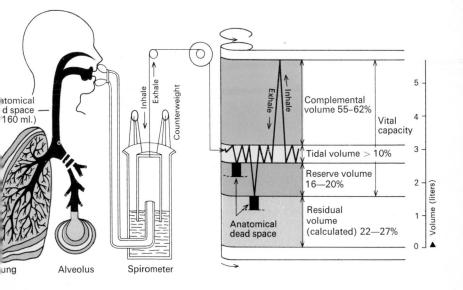

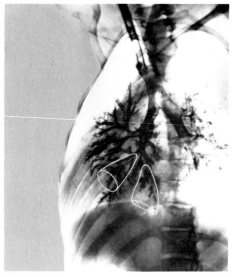

Lung X ray, produced by methods described in the text, reveals bronchiectasis (widening of the bronchi after chronic infection) in two bronchopulmonary segments, whose cone-like shapes are superimposed. Remainder of the bronchial tree shows a more normal pattern. Bronchiectasis is difficult to eradicate other than by surgery, and such X rays show precisely which parts need to be dealt with.

pattern; but note that the tidal volume is near normal and in its right place. In other words the patient's chest is not always near its maximum expansion. The result is that—except during exertion—the patient has no symptoms. But even moderate effort can bring on breathlessness and rapid breathing over the full range of the again restricted vital capacity.

These are "perfect" cases. In real life they can lie closer together in spirometer tests than these descriptions indicate. One further test can help to clarify the nature of the condition. The operator asks the patient to inhale deeply and to breathe out as fast as he can. This reveals the rate of the breathing cycle. Results are shown in the lower graphs in the same diagram. Asthma patients will breathe in normally, out much more slowly—so that a maximum 30 per cent, say, of their vital capacity is exhaled in one second. (This is called the forced expiratory volume in one second, or FEV1 for short; a healthy person's FEV1 is 80 per cent of his vital capacity.) Patients with emphysema or edema will have an FEV1 of 80 or even 85 per cent of their (much reduced) vital capacity.

Such tests can tell us what is wrong with the lungs but not where the seat of the trouble lies, for only rarely is the condition uniformly spread throughout the lungs. Where this issue cannot be decided by obvious techniques (listening down a stethoscope;

tapping the chest to locate dull, airless parts of the lung; looking down the trachea with a bronchoscope or listening down it with microphones; and so on) we turn to studies with X rays and radioactive gases.

For X-ray studies we do one lung at a time so that in side view the passages made visible are not superimposed. To do the left side, for instance, we lie the patient on his left and, after locally anesthetizing his throat and larynx, push a soft rubber catheter down into his trachea and pour through it about 10 ml. of iodized oil (lipiodol), which is radio-opaque. Within minutes the oil spreads to coat the trachea and the bronchi and we can take X rays like the one shown opposite.

If the trouble lies in the bronchioles or alveoli, we use an atmosphere in which all the gases are normal except that some of the nitrogen is replaced by a radio-isotope of the rare gas xenon. Scintillation counters on the chest reveal which parts of the lung this atmosphere is failing to penetrate or areas where it is present in abnormal volumes. We can also take readings over a blood vessel in an arm or leg, to see how effectively the labeled gas passes into the blood through the alveolar membrane.

Tests of Heart Function

Except during major surgery the heart is so inaccessible and so well protected that we must conduct most of our tests at some distance from it. We have already studied the EKG, which, you will remember, can tell us plenty about the shape of the heart, the regularity of its rhythm, and the condition of its muscle and conducting system, but very little about its output, or the state of its valves and internal walls or septa (unless defects in these members have produced secondary changes in the muscle).

The best external indicators of failure in the valves and septa are the sounds the heart makes. And the best way to hear those sounds is to put your ear straight on the chest wall. The normal heart makes a double beat that can be transcribed phonetically as *lub-dup*—in other words, the first sound is softer and longer than the second. The origin of these sounds is shrouded in erudite controversy, which it would be fruitless to explore here. What is certain is that the "lub" coincides with the contraction of the ventricles and the "dup" comes immediately after the almost simultaneous closing of the aortic and pulmonary valves. A third sound, like a rapid echo of the "dup," is normal in young adults. And a fourth sound, related to atrial contraction, can be heard with electronic aids (and, some claim, by the naked ear). If any of the valves or septa leak or if a valve is too narrow, then either the normal sounds will be modified or extra noises and murmurs will creep in. The timing of these extra sounds and their exact location on the chest wall give a clue to the nature of the fault and to which valve or septum is affected.

The Phonocardiograph

The location is often easier to find with a stethoscope than with the naked ear. The phonocardiograph (PKG) illustrated on page 86 is an elaboration of the stethoscope. Something of a mystique has grown around this machine and exaggerated claims from some users come dangerously near to obscuring its real value in diagnosis. The PKG gathers no *more* information than the humble stethoscope. This is not the same as saying it is no more valuable than the stethoscope; it displays the information in an objective form that can be analyzed and discussed and it provides a record against which the success of surgery or other therapy can be gauged. A further advantage is that we can record several parts of the heart and the arterial and venous pulses in the neck simultaneously and display them all alongside an EKG.

The chart on page 86 is an idealized PKG recording matched with jugular and carotid pulses and an EKG. The diagram is intended merely to show the normal synchronization of events in these four traces. In actual PKG's there are at least 2 PKG traces, often recorded through different frequency filters, and the arterial and venous pulses are rarely recorded simultaneously. We use the jugular venous pulse as a guide to events in the right side of the heart and the carotid arterial pulse when investigating the left side. Below the chart you can see the regions of the PKG associated with valve defects.

The PKG is more useful for diagnosing valve defects than septal defects, particularly small ones. To measure septal defects accurately we have to enter the heart by cardiac catheterization.

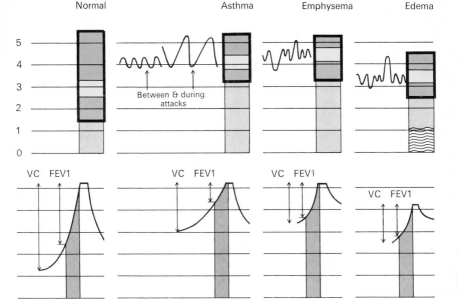

| Normal | Asthma | Emphysema | Edema |

Between & during attacks

VC FEV1   VC FEV1   VC FEV1   VC FEV1

Abnormal breathing patterns associated with various conditions are shown in the top row of charts—each of which reads from right to left. Compare them with the normal patterns on page 81 (summarized in upper left histogram). In each histogram the vital capacity is bounded by a black line. The lower charts were made by asking the patient to breathe in fully and let out his breath as fast as possible. The gray bars mark a one-second interval and define the forced expiratory volume in one second (FEV1). VC stands for vital capacity. The text examines these charts in greater detail.

The spirometer at right consists of a tube and bellows. It records the forced expiratory volume in one second (FEV1) and the vital capacity, on a dial instead of on a moving chart. The same make of machine is shown with its back to the camera.

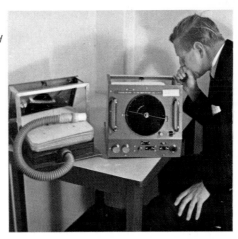

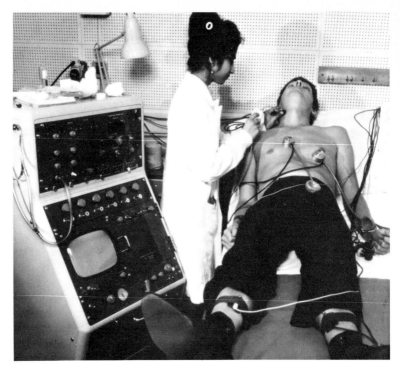

▶ Seconds

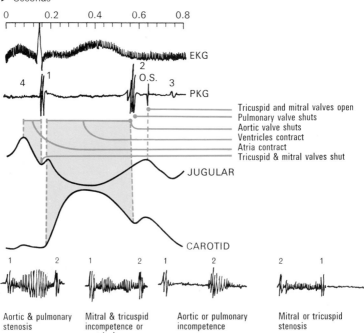

Tricuspid and mitral valves open
Pulmonary valve shuts
Aortic valve shuts
Ventricles contract
Atria contract
Tricuspid & mitral valves shut

EKG
PKG
JUGULAR
CAROTID

Aortic & pulmonary stenosis

Mitral & tricuspid incompetence or ventricular septal defect

Aortic or pulmonary incompetence

Mitral or tricuspid stenosis

Cardiac Catheterization

This highly specialized (and, in unskilled hands, risky) technique has recently played a great part in the study of congenital heart abnormalities, in diagnosing heart disease accurately and objectively, as a prelude to surgery, and in correlating heart output with other physiological changes in the body. The catheter itself is a radio-opaque nylon tube between 1 and 4 mm. in diameter, depending on its purpose. It is pliable and has a slightly curved end so that by rotating it the tip can be lined up with the various orifices through which it must be guided.

Children are often catheterized under general anesthetic, but with adults only a local anesthetic is needed. For catheterization of the right (venous) side of the heart the physician exposes a vein in the right arm and inserts the catheter, and immediately injects heparin to prevent clotting. The catheter, filled with saline to prevent air from entering the blood, is then pushed up the vein until it reaches the superior vena cava, one of the large veins that drain directly into the heart. At frequent intervals the physician checks the course of the catheter on a fluoroscope—a low-dosage X-ray screen whose weak image is electronically intensified before it is displayed. The X-ray dosage to the patient is recorded on a cumulative meter and documented.

From here the physician can move the catheter down into the inferior vena cava to make readings of the kind shown on page 47, or he can go directly into the right side of the heart. There he can take pressure readings by connecting the catheter directly to a pressure recorder, or do PO_2 determinations by withdrawing samples of blood from the catheter. Since the catheter is moving in the same direction as the blood, he can enter the right ventricle and even go out into the pulmonary artery. If he works the catheter up this artery until it wedges in one of its branches, he

The photograph opposite shows a patient and machine rigged for a PKG. Two microphones are held to the greased chest by suction and the technician is taking the patient's venous pulse in the neck using a sensitive barometer probe. The machine is recording on internal photographic paper—hence no display on the oscilloscope. An EKG is also being recorded. The diagram is an idealized phonocardiogram compared with EKG and pulse waves in jugular vein and carotid artery. The labels identify key events in the cycle. 1, 2, 3, and 4 are the heart sounds; O.S. is the "opening snap" (so called) of the mitral and tricuspid valves. Below are shown typical aberrations of the normal PKG and the conditions associated with them (a valve with stenosis is too narrow to let blood pass easily; an incompetent valve is one that leaks).

Normal	Atrial septal defect	Ventricular septal defect	Patent ductus arteriosus

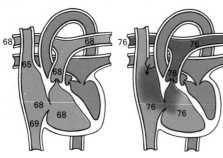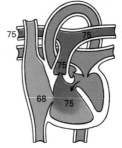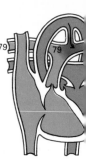

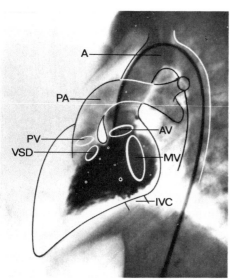

Shown above are percentage saturation of oxygen readings obtained during cardiac catheterization of the right side of one healthy and three defective hearts. These readings provide a basis for calculating the severity of the defect.

Angiogram shows a hollow catheter passing up the aorta (A), through the aortic-valve orifice (AV), and into the left ventricle. Radio-opaque medium from the catheter fills the ventricle. Some has leaked through a ventricular septal defect (VSD) into the right ventricle—hence its abnormal occurrence in the pulmonary artery (PA). Outlines are superimposed to aid clarity. Pulmonary valve (PV), mitral valve (MV), and inferior vena cava (IVC) are also shown.

can record the pressure in the left atrium as it is transmitted back through the lung capillaries. And if there is a septal defect he can pass the catheter through into the left side of the heart and make further readings there.

To study the flow of blood he can inject radio-opaque dyes into any part of the heart and take cine (24/sec.) or rapid still (6/sec.) X-ray pictures of its course. And if for some reason the X-ray dosage would be inadvisable, he can get an approximate picture of circulation defects by injecting a dye and monitoring its circulation and the speed with which it is diluted. Diagrams and pictures on these pages show some results obtained by cardiac catheterization.

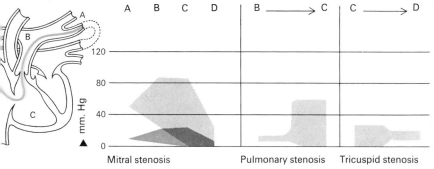

	A	B	C	D	B $\longrightarrow$ C	C $\longrightarrow$ D

Mitral stenosis   Pulmonary stenosis   Tricuspid stenosis

Blood-pressure abnormalities associated with various valve defects are shown above (normal in darker gray). Pressures are taken through the catheter (green) at four points: A—pulmonary wedge pressure, which is equivalent to left atrial pressure (see text); B—pulmonary artery pressure; C—right ventricular pressure; D—right atrial pressure.

Angiogram of right side of heart shows a hollow catheter passing up the inferior vena cava and through the tricuspid-valve orifice into the right ventricle. Radio-opaque medium, passed into the ventricle through the catheter, is ejected through a stenosed pulmonary valve. Above the valve the artery is dilated due to the jet and its associated turbulence. (Normal outline shown.)

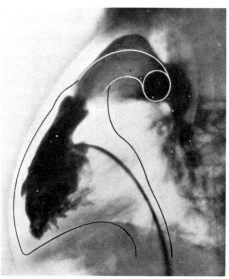

The left side of the heart is more difficult to catheterize. The physician is working against the bloodflow the whole way—and the pressure is much greater on the arterial side. To enter the left ventricle he has to choose the moment when the aortic valve is open. If he mistimes it, he can tear or damage the valve; if he aligns the tip wrongly, he can go into a coronary artery. Similar dangers attend the passage (also against the valve movement) from the left ventricle into the left atrium. But I do not want to create an oversimplified picture in your mind: right side, child's play; left side, tiger country. The right side has its dangers too— particularly when the physician is trying to guide the tip through a hole in the septum so as to get readings of the left side. From the right atrium one slip could push the catheter out through the heart wall, or through the septum, or across a coronary artery, or into the coronary sinus or the aorta, or tearing through the tricuspid valve, or through the atrio-ventricular node—one of the key parts of the conducting system.

In short, catheterization can be highly risky. In its early days and in places still today, it was and is indulged in for its own sake, with meager returns in diagnosis compared with other, safer methods. After all, what does it matter whether a patient has aortic stenosis with mitral regurgitation or aortic regurgitation with mitral stenosis? Either way he's going to need open-heart surgery. True, catheterization would clinch it, but once the heart is open the information, gained at such risk, becomes superfluous. The surgeon can then see the trouble with his own eyes. As Lord Brock, a great surgeon, once said: "The cold white light of surgery is a better diagnostic tool than the cardiac catheter." (Also—referring back to heart sounds—he once said, at a meeting in which the physicians were getting a bit precious about the opening snaps and ejection clicks they claimed to hear: "The heart is a pump, not a damned musical box!")

By dealing with the vital functions in sequence I have inevitably diminished any sense you might have of their interconnection. To reestablish that sense let us round off this account by imagining one fault at one point in the system and seeing how it affects everything else. Our patient has, let us say, mitral-valve stenosis and regurgitation. To squeeze blood into the left ventricle through this stenosed valve his left atrium must work harder; its internal pressure rises. The left ventricle must work harder, too, because some of the blood it pumps regurgitates back through the mitral valve. The ventricle grows slightly bigger. The regurgitating blood adds enormously to the left atrial pressure; soon the atrium cannot cope with these large pressures and, instead of pumping, it begins to fibrillate—that is, its muscle fibers contract at random instead of in concert. The effect spreads to the right atrium, which also fibrillates. This poses a severe problem for the right ventricle: it does not get primed properly and it has to work, through the lung network, against the large back-pressure in the left atrium. The right ventricle enlarges greatly.

Because the capillary pressure is increased, the patient's lungs develop edema. They become stiff and inefficient and there are occasional hemorrhages. The venous pressure rises, too, because the right atrium is no longer pumping. This damming-back effect damages the liver, because the pressure gradients through its tissue are not steep enough. The same is true throughout the body: the arterial pressure is high enough to force serum out of the capillaries, but the venous pressure is not low enough to let the serum back into the bloodstream. The sodium-pump mechanism in the cells becomes less effective in these circumstances, and, because the Na^+ ions attract water, the tissues become waterlogged.

To cope with this the doctor gives the patient a diuretic to stimulate kidney action and get rid of the water. Unfortunately the kidneys inevitably excrete potassium under such stimulus. The patient becomes K^+ depleted and his muscles—particularly those of the heart and gut, which are constantly at work—grow less efficient. As a result there is a general lowering of circulatory efficiency. The patient is now on a downward spiral that only surgery can reverse—if his doctor refers him for surgery at the proper time.

Almost every machine discussed so far in this book would detect these defects. The enlarged right ventricle would show in the EKG as a change in the heart's electrical axis. Cardiac catheterization with pressure readings and angiography would show the site and severity of the heart damage. The stenosed mitral valve would show in a PKG. The lung edema would give a reduced vital capacity in spirometer readings. The hemorrhages and other lung damage would show in an X-ray plate. Samples of blood chemicals would reveal the liver damage. And the kidney's K^+ excretion would be detected in urine samples.

All of which demonstrates, once again, the colossal and dynamic unity of our system—something that such labels of convenience as "mitral-valve stenosis" or "pulmonary edema" all too readily disguise.

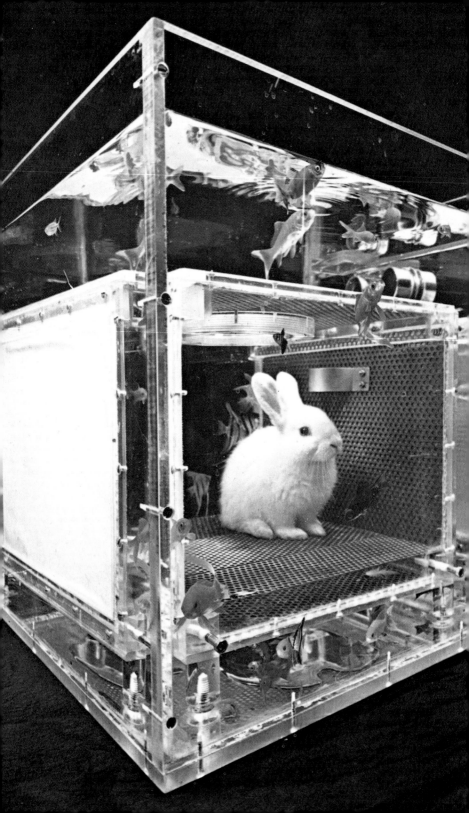

5 Therapeutic Machines

When we want to assess our present state of progress it is often helpful to compare it with our goal, some imaginary ultimate state. In the field of machines it usually turns out that science fiction writers get there before the rest of us. (The most famous case is the prediction by Arthur C. Clarke of communications satellites in stationary orbit over the equator; he made it 17 years before the first such satellite, *Telstar*, was orbited and at a time when most professional scientists would have put the achievement 50 years away.)

I am not a science fiction addict myself, but I asked friends who are, to search their shelves and see what they could find. It was a bizarre and entertaining collection. My two favorites were: (1) a DNA reader that could rebuild a patient according to his genetic blueprint—much as you might rebuild a badly neglected vintage car from the maker's original specifications; and (2) a bottle full of fine powder, each grain of which was a micro-machine: liberated into the bloodstream, these billions of machines, each with a specialized function, would visit every part

This rabbit is completely surrounded by water but is breathing oxygen passing through the membrane-covered sides of its Perspex cage. The membrane, a man-made silicone rubber called polydimethylsiloxane, *has the remarkable property of being able to transport oxygen and carbon dioxide in a way comparable to the physiological action of the alveolar membrane in the lungs. Its breathability makes it highly suitable for use in oxygenators of heart-lung machines, which could be made much smaller than at present. As this chapter states, this and similar membranes could be the basis of many different types of therapeutic machines.*

of the body and tend it, much as an army of gardeners tends a large public park, repairing the ravages of visitors, pests, and time.

Biologically speaking these two fantasies are both near and wide of the mark. They are near in realizing that disease and disorder are cellular phenomena; but they are wide in the analogies they choose (vintage-car restorer and gardener). The second, in particular, forces us to realize that the body already has millions of such "gardeners"—the repair and defense tissues we have evolved over the last 2000 million years or so. Any worker who sets out to compete with these tissues is courting failure.

But, realizing this, we can define our true goal more tightly. It must surely be to design machines that aid the natural action of these repair and defense tissues. Even this tightly defined goal is far beyond our grasp at present.

The most elaborate machines in this category—heart-lung machines, kidney machines, and respirators—were described at length in Chapter 3 of *Spare-Part Surgery*, so a detailed description here would be out of place. Nevertheless, in the light of my present argument, it is worth picking out some of the points I made in that chapter, before looking in detail at recent progress.

The Heart-Lung Machine

The heart-lung machine (photograph on page 97) is a large and complex machine that can barely support a motionless, supine patient. It maintains arterial pressure high enough to nourish his brain and his deeply relaxed tissues, as well as to keep his kidneys active. The machine also maintains the blood PO_2 and PCO_2 at appropriate levels. To do this it needs the constant vigilance of one technician in the steady state and another whenever changes have to be made. Despite all our care it handles the blood so roughly that it can be used on any one patient for only a few hours; our hopes of using it to allow ailing hearts or lungs to rest and recuperate are as distant as ever. This $6000+ machine could not support a man during moderate exertion (ignoring, for present purposes, difficulties over securing the tubes and ensuring partial anesthesia). If the man followed a rigid program of work, so that his precise requirements at each instant could be worked out in advance, three skilled technicians could just about meet those requirements by manipulating the machine; but even then an intelligent homunculus in the blood-stream would know that things were not quite normal. It would notice, for instance, that a lot more red blood cells than usual were being destroyed—that is, more than the normal 1000 per second. More important, it would notice that blood protein was being denatured. This denaturing is due partly to direct contact with O_2, partly to strong shearing forces set up when disks spin or bubbles rise through the blood. In short, these machines are unresponsive to the patient's needs, unwieldy to use, and unacceptably damaging except for brief spells. These disadvantages define two areas in which we must seek improvements.

The first concerns the physical characteristics of the machine. It must handle blood without causing hemolysis and without denaturing its protein. Coupled with this the total blood-handling volume, or prime, of the machine must be made much smaller—or, to put it another way, the efficiency of gas exchange per unit volume of blood must be increased. The best modern machines have a volume around 1 liter—small enough to enable us to prime them with sterile plasma-like fluids without diluting the patient's blood too much. Others, with volumes greater than 1.5 liters, must be primed with bottled blood, which has the attendant dangers of infection, particularly jaundice, and sensitization to serum proteins (an immune response) and to minor blood groups. We must bring the prime down to 0.5 liter, at which level we could use such small volumes of sterile fluid, or even the patient's own blood, that we should avoid the risks of dilution, infection, and sensitization.

The second area covers the control of these machines. The control parameters are all fairly easy to measure: arterial and venous pressures, blood temperature, blood-flow rate, and blood-gas tensions. Pressures, temperatures, and flows are displayed on the machine; gas tensions are measured from time to time on a machine like the one illustrated on page 56—chiefly to determine PCO_2, since PO_2 is fairly clear from the color of the blood in the return lines. In principle there is no reason why these measurements should not be homeostatically linked directly to the controls and so enable the machine to maintain any chosen steady state. Why have we not done so? The obvious answer is that heart-lung machines are used in tricky situations, when the effects of mismanagement—even slight mismanagement—could be fatal. Also there could be numerous changes between one steady state and the next, so the technicians would spend more time controlling the machines than would the homeostats. Nevertheless the fundamental reason for the lack of autoregulation is tied in with the machines' biological unsuitability. Nobody connected with the development of heart-lung machines is happy with the present state of the art. In a despairing moment I have called them a string of blood-smashing devices in series with a protein-denaturing attachment. Nevertheless they allow highly skilled and specialist surgeons to undertake major cardiac operations with remarkably good results.

The kind of machine we really need is a little box that we can put on supports over the patient's stomach. It will have two knobs—one for flow, one for temperature; and it will be worked by the surgeon himself or one of his assistants. It will be so gentle that it will neither call for a large team to manage it nor force the surgeons to be hasty. Emergency support for a coronary victim could even be performed by any competent surgeon in the patient's own home.

It turns out, then, that the two areas in which we must strive for improvements are intimately related. It simply is not worth trying to autoregulate present-day machines. But if we can get one that is small and gentle enough to overcome the physiological objections to existing monsters, it will be eminently worthwhile to build in a high degree of autoregulation.

Such a machine must be built around a breathing membrane that allows O_2 and CO_2 to dissolve in it and then to pass through. By preventing direct contact between gaseous O_2 and blood, the membrane makes it impossible for the O_2 and bubble-centered forces to denature the blood proteins. The membrane also allows the blood circuit to be "closed"; present machines are "open" in the sense that the level of the blood in the oxygenator part of the circuit can rise and fall independently of the patient's blood volume. Surgeons may object to this arrangement. "What about

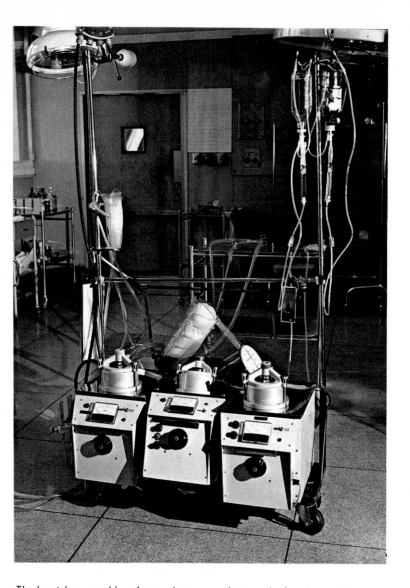

The heart-lung machine shown above can take over the functions of the heart by maintaining arterial pressure at a sufficiently high level for normal functioning of all the patient's organs, and of the lungs by maintaining the appropriate balance of oxygen and carbon dioxide in arteries and veins. It is, however, relatively inefficient in terms of gas exchange per unit volume of blood, and does cause some hemolysis (destruction of red cells). The prototype on page 105 shows how a suitable membrane could act as pump and oxygenator at the same time, with a reduction in the hemolysis rate.

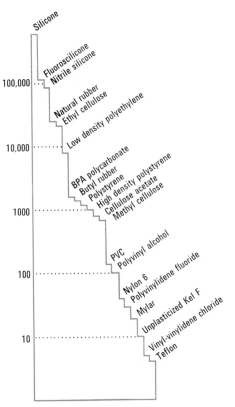

The histogram at left shows the relative permeability of various polymer membranes to O_2. The silicones easily top the list, with biologically unsuitable materials such as rubber and cellulose second. The next best man-made polymers are a whole order of magnitude poorer than the silicones; and even strengthened silicones (fluoro- and nitrile) are far less permeable than the pure (but weak) product. A membrane's permeability to a gas is a product of the solubility and diffusion rate of that gas in the membrane material. The graphs at right show relative diffusion rates and solubilities of a number of materials for O_2 and CO_2. Diffusion rate is closely related to molecular diameter (some gases with diameters between those of O_2 and CO_2 are listed at the base of the first graph). Solubility is closely related to the boiling point of the gases when liquefied. The combination of silicone's fairly flat diffusion-rate graph and elevated CO_2 solubility allows it to breathe CO_2 about six times more effectively than O_2.

blood spilled and leaked during surgery?'' they will ask. "That must surely be sucked away and returned to the circuit for debubbling." The answer is that surgeons must learn not to spill blood. We have experimentally transplanted hearts and lungs for years without spilling blood. We don't even *have* a sucker.

This closing of the circuit will remove the danger that can arise when, for instance, the surgeon inadvertently leans on or moves the venous lines, which drain blood from the patient; this makes the input to the machine fall below its output, and the level of blood in the oxygenator then falls. This, in turn, could lead to inefficient oxygenation and, at very low levels, it could create a danger of pumping a fatal mixture of air and blood

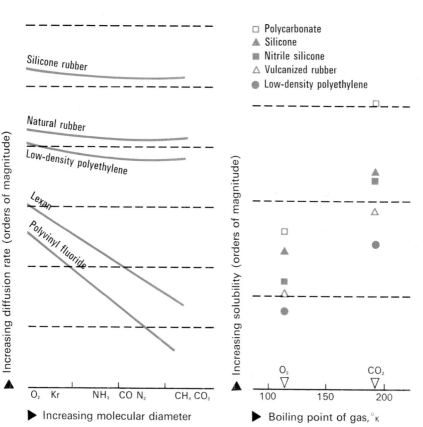

Silicone rubber

Natural rubber

Low-density polyethylene

Lexan

Polyvinyl fluoride

Increasing diffusion rate (orders of magnitude)

O₂ Kr   NH₃ CO N₂   CH₄ CO₂

▶ Increasing molecular diameter

☐ Polycarbonate
▲ Silicone
■ Nitrile silicone
△ Vulcanized rubber
● Low-density polyethylene

Increasing solubility (orders of magnitude)

O₂   CO₂

100   150   200

▶ Boiling point of gas,°ᴋ

into the return line. Everyone who worked on bypass machines in the early days must have had this awful experience at least once. Much of the technicians' time is taken up with the fundamentally unnecessary chore of maintaining adequate levels in the oxygenator. In a closed circuit, the need would vanish.

Finally, if the membranes are designed and stacked in the right way, we can pulse the oxygen to assist the blood flow—perhaps even to the extent of replacing the pumps altogether. Using a gas bubble to massage blood between thin membranes not only creates a gentler form of pump, but also comes closer to the natural oxygenator, the lung. The diameter of the alveolar capillaries is in places as little as 5 microns, so the red cells (average

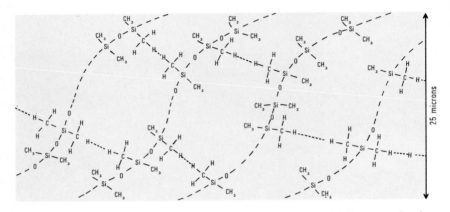

The schematic diagram above shows how the polydimethylsiloxane molecules are considered to be arranged in the membrane. Dashed lines in the chains represent thousands of -Si(CH₃)₂O- groups; dotted lines between chains represent weak hydrogen bonds.

diameter 7 microns) must literally squeeze through in tight contact with the compliant capillary and alveolar membrane; and because each red cell has about 70 times as much oxygen-carrying capacity as the same volume of plasma, this intimate contact greatly enhances gas exchange.

Curiously enough, the ability of the membrane to transport CO_2 is more crucial than its O_2 breathability; the reason becomes clear when we look at the tensions of these gases in the alveoli and their capillaries (see diagram on page 58). The resting PCO_2 in the veins is around 46 mm. Hg; that in the alveoli is around 40 mm. Hg. The gradient across the alveolar/capillary membrane is 6 mm. Hg. Comparable figures for PO_2 are 40 mm. Hg venous and 100 mm. Hg alveolar. The gradient there is 60 mm. Hg—ten times greater. Yet identical quantities of each gas pass in opposite directions each minute—240 ml. In short, the alveolar/capillary membrane is at least 10 times more efficient at transporting CO_2 than at transporting O_2. Actually, from measurements during exertion we know it to be 15 times more efficient, but I illustrate the argument with the resting measurements because they, of course, are relevant to the anesthetized patient.

The charts on pages 98 and 99 show that, on at least two

The membrane can be strengthened by incorporating phenyl or vinyl groups in the polymer as shown at right. These unite molecules of neighboring chains with stronger covalent bonds, but cause a drastic reduction in breathability. The pure membrane is shown below being manufactured in a continuous process at the Royal Postgraduate Medical School in London. Dr. Nora Burns, who has carried out a great deal of research leading to this process, demonstrates the physical appearance of the membrane.

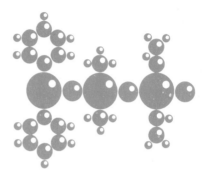

Phenyl
(C₆H₅—)

Methyl
(CH₃—)

Vinyl
(CH₂CH—)

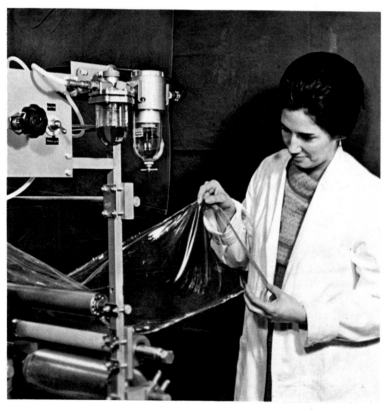

counts, there is only one suitable membrane material: silicone rubber. Not only does it breathe O_2 at least 50 times better than any other plastic, but it also breathes CO_2 at least 6 times more efficiently than O_2—a rare meeting of physiological need and plastics technology. The basic unit for this rubber is the -Si$(CH_3)_2$O- group, which—repeated 7000 to 10,000 times— makes up the polydimethylsiloxane molecule (molecular weight 500,000 to 750,000). The repeated -Si-O-Si-O- backbone imparts flexibility to the molecule (as the diagram on page 100 shows), and the Si-O angle can vary between 140° and 160°. This not only allows the molecule to stretch, but also enables it to twist on its own axis without contracting. This ability had a great deal to do with the permeability of silicone membranes to gases; calculations show that a twisting motion of three -Si-O- units creates an opening in the polymer sufficient to permit a gas molecule to jump through. (The full explanation of this permeability involves calculations of electron density too technical for this discussion, but it is interesting to see that in complexity the mechanism begins to approach some of the simpler physiological processes.)

The pure polymer can be formed into sheets as thin as 12.5 microns (0.0005 inch). Unfortunately it is difficult to handle because it is tacky and develops a high electrostatic charge. Its tear strength is also low. This weakness is inherent in the polymer. The only binding force between the molecules is the hydrogen bond, the weakest bond in polymer chemistry. The sheet can be strengthened by incorporating phenyl or vinyl groups here and there along the polymer (see diagram on page 101); such groups unite the molecules with the far stronger covalent bond. Incidentally, they are present to a small degree, up to 3 per cent, in the "pure" methyl silicone rubber. This addition of yet more phenyl and vinyl groups—say, up to 20 per cent— greatly increases the strength of the polymer but at a colossal sacrifice in breathability (see the chart on page 98). In fact, all attempts to use the membrane have failed on this score. The commercially available silicone polymers breathe so slowly that they need areas as big as 7 square meters to supply O_2 to, and remove CO_2 from, the blood of a full-grown patient. Even if we used this commercial membrane as efficiently as possible with the oxygen-pulsing method already described, the volume of the circuit, including tubes, would be at least 1 liter (compared with up to 3 liters for existing machines).

When we consider the other advantages of membrane pumps (low hemolysis, closed circuit, and low protein denaturing) it would obviously be worth while going ahead with commercially available membrane; but as long as we have before us the tantalizing breathability of the pure membrane, which would reduce the area to a mere 2 square meters and the volume to as little as 540 ml., we are unlikely to pursue anything less suitable. If only the membrane could be strengthened without drastically curtailing its breathability!

All around the world, groups of polymer chemists are tackling this problem, usually in great secrecy. The approach is almost entirely empirical, for in polymer chemistry an ounce of experience is worth a ton of theory. One line of attack is to copolymerize the weak silicone with a strong crystalline molecule such as polycarbonate, in which O_2 and CO_2 are highly soluble (more so, in fact, than in silicone), though less diffusible. The other is to find side groups, or groups that can be substituted for -Si-O- groups here and there, so as to raise the strength without changing the breathability. The chief U.S. center is the Dow Corning Laboratory at Schenectady, N.Y. In Britain, most of the work is being done at the Royal Postgraduate Medical School, Hammersmith, London. The Hammersmith group, who worked on the chemistry (that is, the rubber, filler, solvent, and catalyst) as well as on the mechanics of continuous production, are now producing 12.5-micron sheets of rubber with almost unimpaired breathability and easy handling qualities. Their work has greatly increased our chances of producing a disposable membrane oxygenator of modest dimensions.

My own group has been interested in membrane oxygenators for several years now; in fact, I described a prototype in *Spare-Part Surgery*. Results were disappointing because until recently the only available commercial silicone membrane was 400 microns thick and (for some reason) much stickier than the pure polymer. Also the machine, like many prototypes, was far too intricate.

We are now testing a much simpler version.

The development of a membrane that has almost ideal properties has caught us in an unprepared state. As happens many times in medicine when we desperately need and prepare for a fundamental advance in a particular field (in this case in membrane technology) its realization exposes us as not being as ready to make use of it as we thought. In fact many of the display systems for exposing blood to the membrane that we thought would be adequate have proved inefficient. The reason for this is that the systems fail to mimic the lung and to utilize the remarkable properties of the red blood cells, by failing to bring the bulk of the red cells in apposition with the surface of the membrane.

Most workers in this field turned originally to conventional exchanger systems. We are familiar with exchanger systems in everyday life, such as domestic hot-water radiators and car radiators. These are unenclosed exchangers. Efficiency can be increased by enclosing the tubes of the radiator and blowing air through this enclosure, making a typical tube heat exchanger or calorifier. Those of us who were brought up in the railway era of the steam boiler would describe these in terms of Atlantic- and Pacific-type exchangers using tubes extruded in silicone rubber enclosed in an outer casing. (In the Atlantic system blood flows through tubes surrounded by oxygen; in the Pacific system the blood surrounds tubes containing oxygen.) It was a short step to pulse the oxygen in such a device and to valve the blood to achieve pumping. In some experimental oxygenators made by James Andrew some six years ago we were able to massage blood along the tubes with waves of gas pressure. Although the difficulties of manifolding tubes in these systems are gradually being overcome, it is unlikely that such a complicated way of solving the problem will have any place in the general application of oxygenators to extracorporeal circulation.

Professor Denis Melrose and his team at the Royal Postgraduate Medical School, London, are using tube exchangers in their experimental work on the implanted lung. I have always felt that the permanently implanted mechanical heart, with its power supply problems, would not be a practical proposition in the foreseeable future, but in the field of lung replacements this

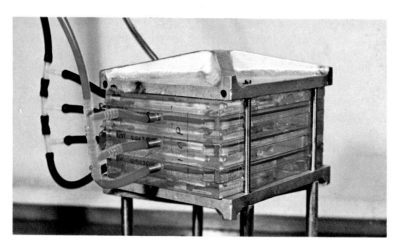

The experimental pump/oxygenator shown above consists of a battery of Perspex and membrane sandwiches. In each of these, blood is massaged between twin membranes as a long bubble of oxygen passes synchronously above and below from the inlet to the outlet slit. Oxygen is delivered in the black tubes. The arrangement of plates and membranes can be seen below. A unit has been dismantled and one membrane drawn back to show the inlet (at the top) and outlet oxygen ports. Using the membrane described in the text this device can oxygenate as much blood as it pumps.

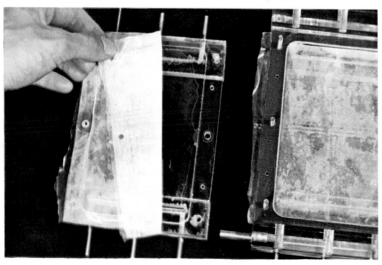

group may achieve a practical mechanical lung before we overcome the special difficulties associated with the transplanted lung. These difficulties are related not to rejection or infection, but to specific substances called *surfactants*. These are detergent surface-active substances that make it possible to inhale air with little effort by reducing the surface tension pull on all the alveoli, which adds up to a considerable force. These substances do not seem to be secreted in a transplanted lung.

There have been two main philosophical approaches in the quest for oxygenators that can be effectively used in bypass surgery. One, the philosophy of expediency, has been to accept low-efficiency devices with a large priming volume so that the benefits of using membranes clinically may be gained immediately; the other, the philosophy of idealism, has been to aim for the highly efficient and ideal compact system. Various "flat-bed" oxygenators are being used tentatively in several centers. The simplest of these consist of pairs of rectangular silicone rubber membrane sheets with blood manifolded in at either end and air or oxygen flowing on the outside of the membranes. Others use disks of membrane with central-to-peripheral blood flow. In these, blood enters through perforations in the middle of the membranes and is led into a manifold through several holes near the periphery of each disk-shaped cell. Piercing the membrane in this way should be avoided wherever possible, however, to prevent leakage of blood with the attendant risks of infection or of gas entering the circulation at these junctions, which are always difficult to seal reliably. These machines fit into the policy of expediency.

Some flat-bed oxygenators are extremely ingenious. One, which has been in clinical use, is made to rock from side to side to achieve turbulence and better blood distribution. This partly overcomes one of the problems encountered in thick blood layers in which all red cells are not in contact with the gas transference membrane as they are in the lung. This results from the natural property of any particulate matter floating or held in suspension in a moving fluid to go to the center of the stream. The supporting fluid forms a boundary layer along the vessel walls and this can be extremely difficult to shift. The rocking oxygenator releases this boundary layer. My gas-pulsing device (shown on page 105) also overcomes this effect to some extent, and many other prototype membrane oxygenators have tackled the problem in different ways. It is interesting to note that the philosophy of expediency has been tried clinically in several forms. The Bramson oxygenator used by the team led by Frank Gerbode in Los Angeles has given the largest experience. This operates on the radial flow principle mentioned earlier, accepting the shortcomings of manifolding through perforations in the membrane. It has been very successful and has obviated some blood damage. The second, nearer the ultimate approach, has been used by the Minneapolis group led by Walter Lillehei, who pioneered the use of the bubble oxygenator. They have now used the pulsed membrane clinically.

There is little doubt that membrane devices will be used as life-support machines to aid a failing heart or lung. Some devices have been developed to reduce the work of the left ventricle very considerably. One works by sucking blood from the main arteries in the groins during the ejection phase of the heart and replacing it under pressure during the filling phase. If this technique is to succeed it presupposes that reliable EKG triggering is available to prevent the device from discharging whilst the heart is ejecting. It also assumes that the mechanism that has evolved over the last few hundred million years to ensure that both sides of the heart put out the same amount of blood with each beat can be violated without causing further damage to the heart. This assumption is probably not valid. The small number of experimental studies of this problem are equivocal. We do not yet know the answer. It is because of these problems that life-support machines for heart or lung failure will eventually be in the form of small membrane pump oxygenators to partly bypass and do the work of both ventricles and the lungs. These will be connected from the large veins in the groins to pump oxygenated blood into the arterial system in the same region.

Another use for small membrane heart-lung machines is for organ storage. They have a greater advantage in this field than in clinical perfusion, for it is here that we have to be even more careful to avoid denaturing proteins. The reason for this is that there are no other organs in the system (such as the liver and kidneys) to mop up and process the products of blood destruction as there are in the complete organism. This has been one of the limiting factors in the formation of organ banks.

The Kidney Machine

One major problem associated with kidney machines is how to maintain correct concentration in the dialyzate. It is worth studying in depth—not because the system is terribly ingenious (in fact, by the standards applied in modern oil refineries it is fairly elementary), but because it highlights the strategy of autoregulation in situations where physiological limits must be very accurately observed.

The problem is this: dialyzate—a mixture of large sugar molecules and ions—is a perfect culture medium for bacteria, especially when warmed to blood temperature before passing through the kidney machine. So we cannot mix and store the large quantities we need (400 liters or more per patient per session). We therefore store the dialyzate as a thin concentrated syrup, which we dilute about 30 times with ordinary tapwater before heating it and passing it through the machine. Syrups are inherently sterile, of course, because their osmotic forces suck any invader dry.

On the face of it, nothing could be simpler than diluting a known concentrate. One of the most satisfactory methods, shown to me four or five years ago by Willem Kolff, the pioneer of kidney machines, is also among the most simple—a sterile glass container, fillable with up to 1 liter of concentrate, and a larger container, fillable with up to 30 liters of tapwater, both of which, when full, automatically discharge into a single tank. As long as the manufacturer works to a precise specification and there is plenty of help around the kidney unit, the method is fine. But humans are expensive and manufacturers can err, so there is a widespread need for an automatic mixer. And that is where the real problems begin.

The obvious way of turning this batch method into a continuous one is the proportioning pump. If the dilution is to be 30 to 1, one cylinder is made 30 times bigger than another, and both discharge into a common outlet. Unfortunately, the dilution is not always 30 to 1. A patient in heart failure, for instance, has a high concentrate of Na $^+$ in his serum and, to reduce it, we dialyze him against a very low Na $^+$ dialyzate—say, 123 mEq/liter. To keep the other constituents normal, the concentrate must be especially made with a low Na $^+$. But—and this is the point—the physician wants to be *sure* he is dialyzing against 123 mEq/liter ± 1 of Na $^+$. In other words, the tolerable variation is less than 1 per cent. It is not that greater variations would harm the patient

One version, which has been used clinically, of the continuous system for diluting dialyzate is shown below. Cold mains water is reduced in pressure and heated to between 15° and 20°C before going into a pump jet aspirator. An electric conductivity cell (ECC) in the mixing tank controls the solenoid needle valve (S1) in the concentrate supply line. At the start the ECC registers the low conductivity of air and the valve is kept fully open. As the ECC becomes covered, it records a high conductivity and the needle closes down. Two pumps operate continuously below the mixing tank. One recirculates the liquid through a de-airer, the other transfers liquid to a header tank. A second ECC monitors the outflow from this tank according to the high and low levels preset on the final conductivity meter. If the conductivity (and hence the concentration) is outside these limits, S6 is opened and the liquid goes to waste. When the concentration of the dialyzate comes within the required range, S6 is closed and S5 is opened. A final monitor warms the dialyzate to body temperature.

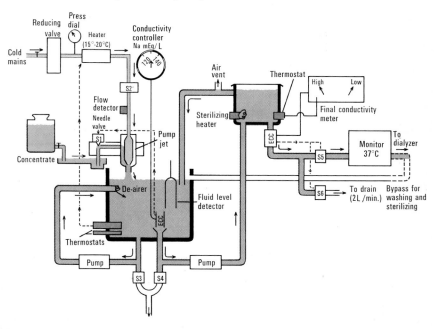

much, but the physician must have a precise base line against which to measure his therapy.

There are several possible sources of error: bubbles in the water, leaking lines, faulty makeup of the concentrate, faulty labeling, faulty selection among correctly labeled concentrates, and (rarely) wear in the proportioning pump. (The bubbles, incidentally, come when the water is heated; cold water has more than 20 ml/liter of dissolved air, but at blood heat has room for only 14 ml/liter. Falling pressure can also fetch out bubbles; they are a nuisance throughout the machine, not just at the pump.) To safeguard against errors, the makers added a conductivity meter to the system. The conductivity of the dialyzate is an accurate measure of its concentration: for instance, if the dilution rises or falls by 1 per cent, the conductivity falls or rises by 1 mho (reciprocal ohm) per cm^3 across the 18-mm. gap of the conductivity electrodes. More problems followed: voltages strayed; meter sensitivities varied with temperature and wandered in time; bubbles that gathered on the electrodes upset the readings. The guard itself needed guarding!

We found the system unsatisfactory for the very accurate dialysis needed by some heart patients. Not that the dilution was inaccurate, but any of the faults I have listed caused the machine to switch itself off and sound an alarm—like a train whose only controls are a start button and an emergency brake. What we wanted was a machine that could accept any inaccuracy in the pump and in the concentration of the concentrate but that, instead of calling for help, could actually *compensate* for these deficiencies. It sounds like a tall order. One's mind instantly flies to elaborate, hierarchical systems of controls and counter-controls. Not a bit. In fact the device we ended up with could hardly be simpler—thanks largely to Philip Allen, development engineer at Allen Die & Tool Co., who developed the machine. My idea was to use a recycle system. The valve, being controlled by a conductivity meter, allowed varying amounts of concentrate into the water—more if the conductivity was low, less if it was high. In short, feedback from the product was used to regulate the quality of the product. We built a breadboard version that proved the scheme was workable. It was at this stage that Philip

Allen became involved. He pointed out at once that the pumps were both costly and irrelevant. And between us we produced the jet-pump system diagramed on page 109. The pump comes free—it belongs to the water company and is at the far end of the water main. By forcing the water through a constriction we get a rise in velocity and a decrease in pressure—enough to aspirate the concentrate into the flow. The tap in the aspirator tube is controlled by a conductivity meter, which varies the amount that can be aspirated and thus controls the dilution. Accuracy is better than 1 per cent. As a double check a second conductivity meter is put in the tank and the circuitry arranged so that environmental changes in temperature and voltage have countervailing effects on the two meters. Thus if supply voltages stray, or ambient temperature changes, or meter sensitivities wander, one meter reads high and the other low; their difference is magnified. The output of both meters is compared in the control box, which can sound an alarm and switch everything off.

The system had an unexpected bonus. The pressure beyond the constriction dropped as low as 50 mm. Hg, at which *all* dissolved air comes out of solution. True, the pressure rises immediately afterwards, but the gas bubbles do not quickly redissolve. Thus we incorporated a swirl in the line, which concentrates the light air bubbles at its center while throwing the heavier water to the periphery. The water beyond the swirl was totally de-aired and despite later heating and pressure gradients, no bubbles could form in the system or the kidney machine. The swirl was the brainchild of Robert Bass, aerodynamics engineer with Dowty Rotol Co., who has worked closely with us on many devices.

The entire machine has only one moving part: the valve in the aspirator line. If you are an engineer you may see nothing particularly remarkable about that. A large part of the modern chemical industry relies on machines in which inlet and outlet valves are the only moving parts, and in which information from the system is the sole means of controlling those valves. It may come as a surprise to learn that this approach to machines is rare in medicine. Doctors (and it is still doctors who design most of the nonelectric medical hardware) tend to think in terms of safe, mentally graspable classical mechanics—of physical enclosure and positive displacement, of guard circuits that, instead of feeding back cybernetically, sound alarms and shut everything down. A good example of this sort of attitude and the opposite approach is the provision of a totally sterile environment.

A Curtain of Air

In the operating theater and recovery room we want, ideally, a bacterial count of zero (ascertained by exposing plates of culture medium, culturing the bacteria that fall upon them, and counting the resulting population). For routine surgery we can accept a count up to 30,000 per square meter per hour (although 1000 is easily achieved). (For comparison, a well-kept home averages 1000 in the spare room to millions in the bathroom and bedroom during dressing and bedmaking; a subway station from 100,000 to astronomical figures, depending on ventilation; a garbage dump millions; and a hospital ward around 2000, but bedmaking puts it up to millions—all per square meter per hour.) But for slow-healing tissue, such as bone, which is very susceptible to infection; for transplant patients, whose immune reaction is suppressed and who are therefore defenseless against bacteria; for accident and burn victims, whose systems are badly disturbed by shock; for premature babies, who lack the defenses of the full-term child—for all these we need to get as close to a zero count as possible. In this context it is worth remembering that in even the best surgical centers in the world the postoperative infection rate is 7 per cent—and that the worst source of infection is often the patient himself. Faced with such demands most doctors think at once of rooms built with special nonporous plasters and concretes, with double airlocks and bacteria-filtered air circulation. Such rooms can be kept perfectly sterile, as long as people are excluded. But no matter how well they are scrubbed and gowned and masked, people drop a steady rain of bacteria. In fact, there is plenty of evidence that a thorough scrubbing, by

The sterile environment machine described in the text is shown opposite. The patient is unaware of any draft as carefully directed streams of sterile air isolate him from infection. As the diagram shows, this airflow is divided into two types. Air from the central vents is directed downward to prevent turbulence from the outer currents and to maintain a flow of sterile air over the patient. The peripheral vents direct curtains of air outward at higher flow rates to form a barrier against migration of microorganisms into the central area. A filter at the air intake isolates particles larger than 5 microns, and the main filter is effective down to 0.3 microns.

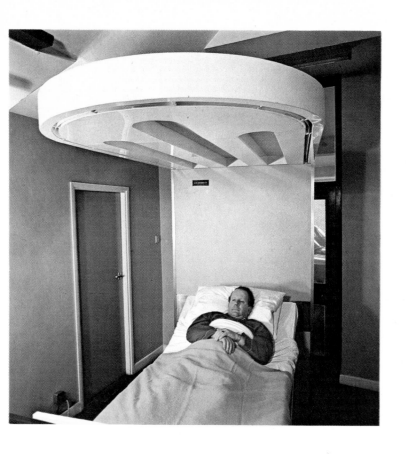

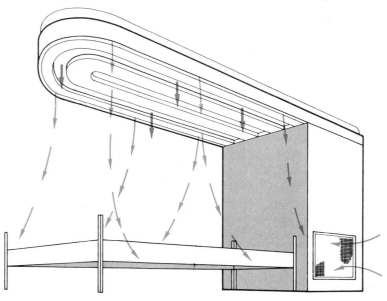

opening the pores, increases this shower of bacteria several thousand per cent.

It is here that techniques used for dust-free assembly of space-craft, airframes, and optical and electronic components have helped. In these industries people realized that you can never get a dust-free room unless you control the air currents in it—in fact, it doesn't matter how much dust there is in the room as long as you can keep a current of pure air flowing over the component. The technique was first applied in medicine in the early 1960s by the bone surgeon John Charnley.

Before we began heart transplantation at the National Heart Hospital, we realized that transplant patients were going to need an ultrasterile environment, especially during the early post-operative stage, when their immune reaction is most heavily suppressed. We had been experimenting for some time with various forms of "air curtaining"—a system in which a gentle downward draft of sterile air (warmed and humidified if necessary) is used in order to maintain a sterile region.

It is very difficult to establish a completely sterile environment. The patient isolation equipment shown below is very effective but there is always the possibility of contamination between sterilizing and erecting the tent.

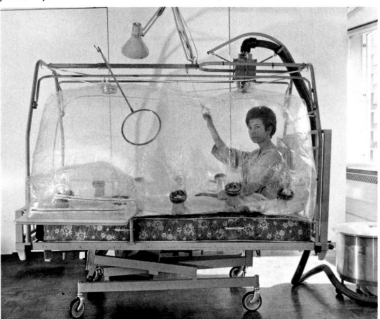

We took our ideas and homemade prototypes to Dr. Douglas Denny, technical director at Bell's Asbestos and Engineering. He simplified the system and developed it up to the point of manufacture. Even he, I believe, was surprised with the result (pictured on page 113); the diagram below shows the air distribution around the bed. The patient, completely unaware of any draft, lies in a *totally* sterile environment—a sterility that even a sideways draft of 14 m/sec cannot intrude upon. The moving air removes bacteria and other pathogens released by the patient (for example, in his breath) and so minimizes the chance of self-infection. Even the inflated polythene tent with fitted gloves, shown opposite, cannot guarantee such perfect sterility, for there is always the possibility of contamination between sterilizing and erecting the tent.

A New Approach

All the developments discussed above are good examples of the benefits that follow when we liberate ourselves from the constraints of what I have called "classical mechanics"—the sort of engineering that has dominated medical machinery to date. It was classical mechanics that produced bubble and disk oxygenators and peristaltic pumps in heart-lung machines, proportioning pumps and guard circuits in dialyzate automixers, and inflated plastic bags with gloves for germ-free environments. I choose these examples because our work has involved me deeply in their development. In each case we began by thinking at a fairly superficial technical level—the level where we talk of improving rather than of redesigning. In each case we were soon forced to abandon such an approach in favor of one that was more fundamental. We had to redefine the role of the machine not in terms of what was technically possible (for as our efforts unfolded we became painfully aware of our ignorance of all the available techniques in all the industries that had, at some time, faced and solved similar problems), but in terms of physiology. In short, we worked outward from the patient and his needs rather than from any particular machine and its capabilities.

In each case, too, that definition of aims is our most significant contribution to the final device; the scientific and engineering contributions came—as indeed they should, but all too rarely do—from scientists and engineers, some of them only partly involved in medicine. I am sure that if my work had led me into other fields, the details of this chapter would have been very different, but the pattern would have been identical. The technology that medicine is now developing and applying is too specialized for doctors alone to manage with ease. In the same way, physiology is too specialized for engineers and chemists to comprehend with the kind of mastery a designer of medical machines must have. The machines we are now contemplating will be a product of both sorts of discipline.

Such machines will be different in kind from present-day products—closer to biology, less obviously mechanical. The membrane oxygenator is a pointer along this route. Living systems operate on seemingly minute gradients; we measure them in *milli*volts, *milli*equivalents, *micro*joules. It is only when we look at the time and distance scale in which these gradients operate that we see how huge they really are. A hundred millivolts across a membrane 75 angstroms thick is equivalent to more than 13,000 volts per centimeter. Yet we have cells within us that can reverse such a polarity more than 500 times in a second. In the laboratory such forces can be highly disruptive—tearing gas molecules apart, vaporizing electrodes, unleashing a storm of electromagnetic radiation. But scale these forces down, as the cell does, and they can be used for the precise transportation of individual molecules. And because the inertia and momentum of individual molecules are vanishingly small compared with the electrical and osmotic forces we can apply, it becomes possible to switch or reverse their motion as rapidly as happens in living cells.

Here we come to the center of biology, for it is the ability to select among individual molecules and ions, to transport them, and to change them, that separates the technology of life from human technology. That is why the membrane oxygenator marks such a radical departure in medical machines. Membranes, of course, are not new, but—like the regenerated cellulose membrane in kidney machines—they have hitherto been passive structures, used as either filters or barriers. The silicone membrane *breathes*; when O_2 and CO_2 move through along their respective pressure gradients, the very molecules of the membrane assist their passage by twisting on their axes. This is not the same thing as active transport, in which molecules and ions are ferried through a membrane against a gradient; yet neither is it totally passive transport, like a kidney machine membrane. It comes in a new category—"assisted passive transport," we might call it. And remember, the polydimethylsiloxane molecule is unknown in nature; it is a product of human ingenuity. Because this membrane works on individual gas molecules very much as living membranes do, it blurs the distinction I have just made between human and living technology. And if we look around at technology in general, we can see many areas in which that same distinction is also breaking down. Metallurgists are growing pure crystal fibers to reinforce alloys. Electronics engineers are doping minute semiconductor layers ("electron membranes," we could almost call them) in order to pack hundreds of components into one square millimeter. Laser experts have developed the ability to produce picosecond (10^{-12} second) pulses of coherent light, pulses only a few wavelengths long; with these they can study chemical reactions whose duration is equally brief—how long before they use the same technique to promote and control new reactions? Biochemists can change individual amino acid units in a DNA strand and study the genetic effects of the changes. Communications engineers can sample several hundred telephone calls thousands of times a second, transmit selected samples down a single cable, sort them out at the receiving end, and turn them back into several hundred seemingly uninterrupted calls. Polymer chemists are developing an increasing ability to make and tailor molecules at will. In short, human technology is beginning to approach the time and distance scales of living technology.

The step from a membrane that can undertake assisted passive transport to one that can actively transport against gradients is conceptionally small—though technologically it is undoubtedly huge. Such membranes must be the basis of future medical machines. Existing machines force upon us methods that are unspeakably crude; we pierce large holes in people (sick people, too), drain off blood, fill them with radioactivity, assault them

118

with giant tubes and catheters, slaughter their cells with X rays and gamma rays, and cut out living samples composed of millions of cells. A selection of active membranes, each designed for a specific set of functions, would allow us to do immeasurably more than we can at present, yet with only the slightest assault on the biological integrity of the patient.

In this context it is not too fanciful to postulate medical "machines" composed entirely of membranous compartments, each filled with a rich soup of biologically active compounds. In some cases they will "live" like parasites in the gut, doing their therapeutic work through the gut wall; in others we shall inject them into muscle (they will be finer than needles and at high velocity their injection will leave marks visible only to high-power microscopy). The feedback element, which all self-regulating machines need, will be part of the chemistry of the membrane. In response to excesses or deficiencies in surrounding fluids, pores will open and ion pumps begin to work, liberating and exchanging chemicals. Whether such machines will be living or dead will be a nice point for philosophers. They will certainly be life-supporting in every way that present-day "life-supporting machines" are not.

If I am right in believing that bio-engineering will make its most fruitful advances along this particular avenue, we are bound to ask how well industry is geared to begin the journey. The answers are all fairly gloomy, I'm afraid.

In medical research it is notoriously easy to raise large university grants for esoteric studies of, for instance, the insolation of human skin in various climates, or blood-group anomalies in isolated rural communities. Yet one might as well bay the moon as ask for modest sums to develop practical machines. That sort of investment, the feeling is, belongs more properly to industry. Such a division ignores the fact that the biomedical machines market is tiny—at the sophisticated end, anyway. A manufacturer recently estimated the total number of heart-lung machines in the world as something under 2000. What scale of research can a market that size support? Other sources—government and agency funds, foundations, and charities—are committee-dominated and unlikely to support large, comprehensive projects.

Who, then, will bring together the production engineers, polymer chemists, biochemists, and doctors? Probably themselves. That is the way things work now and they are unlikely to change. People who want to get things done will seek out people who know how to do them; and between them, somehow, they will manage to divert or beg sufficient money to pay for the work. In a curious way this piecemeal development best suits the anarchic structure of the industry, and will probably prove more effective than the unified-project approach that characterizes Big Science. Perhaps the best thing we can say about the industry is that it has failed to attract big investment. If such investment had come during the last decade, the industry would now be dominated by good managers, obsessed with accountancy and rationalization. They would have thoroughly modernized yesterday's technology. They would plan for tomorrow by extending today's trends.

In this chapter I have shown that tomorrow will not grow out of an improved today. In this field, above all others, there is an increasing need to innovate. Bio-engineers (to lump us all under the one title) must not only be willing to learn things that nobody can now teach them; they must also deliberately unlearn practically everything they have been taught.

Those who are unwilling to change their behavior in this way will lose the race. Let us not forget that at the end of World War II the established radio and electronics firms had excellent managerial reasons for neglecting computers. How could these unwieldy devices, with their thousands of vacuum tubes, miles of wire, and minute data stores, coupled with their huge power drain and acknowledged unreliability . . . how could these ever have any real sales in the everyday business market? Were not the returns in such proven fields as broadcasting and telecommunications much more assured? Only one company had the temerity to question such accountancy—an almost unknown maker of typewriters and adding machines. Its name was IBM.

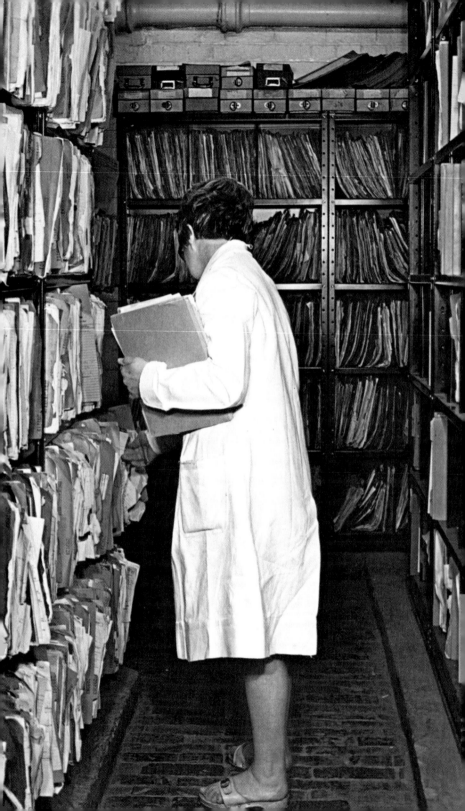

6 Computers and Medicine

After two decades of extraordinarily lusty growth, computers are beginning to approach their infancy. To compound the paradox, they are now in their third generation. This confusion of metaphors aptly characterizes the confusion many people feel when computers first enter their own workaday world. Everybody has seen computers doing wonderful party pieces on TV—designing bridges, composing sound poems, beating junior chess champions, running an entire airline's reservations system, informing politicians on the limits of the possible, and guiding robots infallibly around unknown terrains littered with geometric obstacles. Somehow it is never *those* computers that find their way into one's own industry: somehow one always gets the economy model whose random access store is too small or whose programming language is not quite appropriate to the problem in hand. Nor is that all. The computer's abilities are so idiosyncratic: the intellectual giant that cannot only give you the names and addresses of everyone who bought a given product within the last 12 months, but also list separately those who paid cash, those who used credit cards,

This is the problem facing many hospital records clerks—sorting through shelves of folders in a basement full of shabby hand-written documents to find a case history vital to the treatment of a new patient upstairs. When the doctor has the file he will probably keep it for several hours, during which time it is unavailable to anyone else. The system described on page 142 of this chapter replaces all these documents with a multiaccess computer linked to cathode-ray tube display units that can present the required information almost instantaneously wherever it is needed in the hospital.

those who have since complained, those who live in a certain district—any numerically identifiable category you care to make—this same machine will probably be turned into something worse than moronic by a request to know the amount due from, say, "John Walters, Seaview, 11 King Street," if its file contains only "John Walters, 11 King Street."

This kind of performance, coupled with the unfortunate results of one or two misguidedly ambitious experiments in automation, has hardly helped computers to gain widespread acceptance among doctors. Most doctors react—as indeed most humans react—"There's little I do that a computer could do better, and a lot I do that no computer could do at all." To argue about computers in such terms is to miss the point. In medicine it isn't what men *do* that offers interesting openings for computers, but what they don't do (or can't, or won't). It will be a long, long time before computers are able to substitute for medical man-power in such fields as diagnosis, patient management, or planning the deployment of medical resources. But they are already sufficiently advanced to play other important roles in hospitals and health centers.

First-generation computers had vacuum tubes, small random-access stores, short word lengths, slow computing times. They were essentially off-line machines, suitable for laboratory calculations and payroll accountancy. Second-generation computers had transistors, larger random-access stores, longer word lengths, faster computing times. Many of them were suitable for on-line applications in industry but only the largest and costliest had multiple access for real-time computation. Third-generation computers are built around microminiaturized semiconductors, have large random-access stores, long word lengths, and very fast computing times—all of which has made it possible to provide multiple access to a wide variety of users, each with his own program. And it is this facility that makes the computer an interesting medical machine.

Ninth- or tenth-generation machines (whatever they will be) may replace doctors in some way—in other words, it may by then be possible for a patient to have a direct relationship, in normal language and real time, with a machine. For the moment, though, it is the computer's ability to store, sort, correlate, and perform repetitive tasks—all at an error rate as low as you care to specify—that makes it so valuable.

In the following pages we shall be looking at a computer grid in a fictional group of hospitals. It is based largely on experience in the United Kingdom (chiefly in the United Birmingham Hospitals group), where medicine is centrally organized and such local grids easier to establish than, say, in the U.S.A. Computer applications in the U.S.A., reflecting the individualistic organization of medicine, have concentrated more on particular fields—from the running of individual hospitals or large outpatient departments to the automated interpretation of EKG rhythm disturbances. A lot of fundamental work—on economical coding of medical terms, for instance—has also been done in the United States; such work is, of course, vital if we are to make the best use of computers. But the enormous and surprising benefits we are about to study can most easily come about where there is a common hospital administration for whole regions and where the patients belong to a common scheme or pool.

The system described here does not yet exist (as far as I know) anywhere. But any hospital group that started computing in the early 1960s ought to have achieved it by the early 1970s; it has long been technically feasible—the achievement is more a matter of organization, capital, and will. Every system in the following description already exists, either routinely or as a pilot project, somewhere. The only element of fantasy lies in having brought them all under one roof. By the time this book is published even that may have hardened into fact.

Our hospital—let us call it Boole's Memorial Hospital—is one of a group of eight in a medium-size city; they share a large central computer (hereafter called "center") and its data store. Depending on size each hospital has one or more small computers (hereafter called "local") and a local data store; Boole's has two small computers. Local 1 handles all communications between the hospital and center, and maintains a local store library of current inpatients, and of outpatients due at the next clinic; all other data is in center store (see diagram on page 124). Thanks to this arrangement the hospital could run autonomously

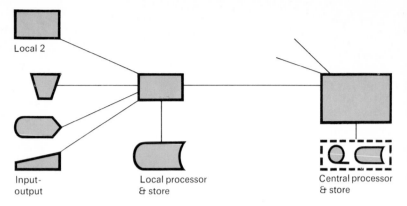

Local 2

Input-
output

Local processor
& store

Central processor
& store

Interfacing of local and central hardware is block-diagramed above. Local processor and store is local 1. Its inputs and outputs include local 2 (which handles requests for services), card readers, display terminals, and keyboards. Having its own store, it can operate autonomously if the central processor is not available. The central system acts as an archive and as a more powerful mathematical machine than the locals.

if communications were severed or center broke down. Local 2 works exclusively between local 1 and the service departments; these include the clinical biochemistry laboratory, EKG, EEG, X-ray, ear-nose-throat, respiratory, and other departments.

Most Boole's inpatients come in from waiting lists generated by the outpatient clinics. For these there is plenty of time to retrieve past records, diagnoses, notes, and summaries. If the patient was treated at another hospital, there is time to send for the relevant documents; if time is short, center can regenerate the documents from data in its store and no physical transfer between hospitals need occur. With emergency admissions it is less easy to match present with past records. The problem is gravest with cardiac patients admitted in heart failure; their past records are often essential to proper treatment. True, most of them carry their name and address, but people marry and divorce, move house, and change their names—all of which can reduce a certainty match to a probability match. If the patient's name is Smith and his address is new, the probability of a match is no better than about 65 per cent in most of England; if computers are ever to be involved directly in clinical work, we shall want probabilities better than 99.9 per cent.

Nevertheless the vast majority of inpatients are correctly registered—as, of course, they were before computers appeared. One big problem in those days was that the data was degraded in use—

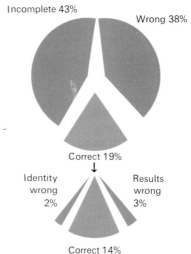

Incomplete 43%

Wrong 38%

Correct 19%

Identity wrong 2%

Results wrong 3%

Correct 14%

Characteristic pattern of errors in the two-way traffic of cards and samples between wards and biochemistry laboratories in a noncomputerized hospital is diagramed at right. Of cards from the wards 43% were correct but incomplete: 38% were wrong—usually in a minor detail like the patient's age or second name. Of the return traffic 10% (or 2% of the total) had results wrongly matched and 15% (or 3% of the total) had them wrongly recorded. The computer system is designed to minimize such errors by handling the laborious tasks (copying names, words, ages, etc.) to a computer, leaving only the key parts (such as recording results) to humans.

particularly where subsequent documents were handwritten, as the diagram above shows. The results depicted there are characteristic of all hospitals where requests are handwritten. There is little chance that the errors and omissions will prejudice the patient's treatment; even requests void of all detail except the patient's surname can be correctly returned—someone at the receiving end is certain to say, "Oh that's Nurse Robinson's handwriting; it must be from Ward 3. Send it back there." The computer, of course, cannot turn detective in this way.

To overcome degradation of this kind, larger hospitals adopted a variation of the stereotype-address system—a malleable metal blank punched with the patient's data, which could be printed onto any document. This system, which dates back to the 1930s in the United States, is now fairly widespread in the world. The computerized system uses the same principle: a master from which any number of duplicates can be generated. Let us look at it first from the point of entry of one particular patient.

A Case History

He is an emergency admission, the victim of a car accident. A passing doctor got to him quickly and noticed, among other things, that his pulse was very slow—about 30 per minute. Is this because the victim is epileptic? or because of damage to his brain (he has a cut forehead)? or because of a heart block? Only hospital tests can tell. All the doctor can do is to give him cardiac massage on the street and in the ambulance. His pulse is still 30/min. on arrival. In the casualty department he is laid slightly head down to maintain the brain circulation and the cardiac massage is stopped because it has no effect. They take a blood sample, which they divide into 4: one for immediate grouping, one for a red-cell count, one for biochemical tests of electrolytes, and one for immediate blood-gas analysis. They notice that the head wound seems superficial and they also spot a scar from an old abdominal operation. Perhaps the operation was done at one of the city's hospitals? If so, his records must be on file at center. It is at this point that the computer becomes involved.

They search his pockets for some identification. Alas, a passing pickpocket was even quicker than the doctor. All they find is an empty envelope with the single handwritten name Vivian Van Leeuwenhoek. It is an office memo holder, so there is no address, stamp, or date. And ambiguity is heightened by the fact that Vivian is a woman's name as well as a man's. (Of course I am making this case as difficult as possible, because only at these limits do we see the full value of the computer's faculty for total recall of any data in its store.) They also find some unidentified pills, which strengthen the epileptic-or-cardiac theories; it would be nice to analyze or identify the pills, but manpower is too scarce on this particular day.

While Van Leeuwenhoek? is being X-rayed, the Boole's register clerk is trying to retrieve any previous records on him. Through local 1 the clerk asks center if any such name is on file. Center replies that it has records of a VIVIAN VANLEEUWENHOZ. (The Z is a code to warn human readers that the surname has more than 13 letters; to save space only 13 fields in the punch card are allotted to the surname, because in Britain only 1 surname in 10,000 is longer than 13 characters. For economy, too, all spaces like the one after VAN are omitted, together with hyphens and apostrophes.) The clerk asks center to type out the categories under which data for VANLEEUWENHOZ are filed.

Center replies: Abdominal, cardiac, and limb fracture. The clerk telephones the casualty doctor and asks which categories interest him. The doctor says that the limb fracture is unlikely to be relevant but the abdominal and cardiac entries may be. The clerk asks center for the summaries under the entries. After a short pause center replies that the data have been dormant for more than five years; they will take 30 or more minutes to retrieve. (Center is programmed to sort through its tapes once a month and weed out any data that have not been recalled during the previous five years. These are transferred onto archive tape and stored in the basement.)

About 35 minutes later—before the patient's X-rays are through—the abdominal and cardiac summaries on VANLEEU-WENHOZ are printed out on the Boole's lineprinter. The abdominal summary is interesting; reading between the lines it becomes clear that almost 8 years ago somebody made a mistake. VANLEEUWENHOZ was admitted to another hospital in the group, with an abdominal pain. Later events make it clear that his was, in fact, a coronary attack. An EKG at the time would have revealed it but, for some reason, no EKG was taken and VANLEEUWENHOZ was opened up for a suspected inflamed gall bladder. No inflammation was found and he was sewn up again; the pain, by coincidence, cleared up, and he was discharged. Some 2 years later, the cardiac summary shows, he had another coronary event—correctly diagnosed this time—followed by a temporary heart block.

The letter in his pocket, the abdominal scar, the present heart block, and the pills—all these make it close on certain that VANLEEUWENHOZ, Van Leeuwenhoek, and the accident victim are one and the same person. Thanks to the rapid retrieval of his past history, the doctors at Boole's can now act appropriately. They take him up to the cardiac unit, where they put him on a slow intravenous drip containing isopropylnorepinephrine, a hormone that stimulates nerve and muscle activity. His pulse soon rises to a safer 38 to 40/min. and he becomes semiconscious.

The X rays show no skull fracture, but his heart is slightly larger than normal. His blood pressure, too, is high—210/30 as opposed to 120/80 for normal adults. Since the summary of the cardiac event 6 years back makes no mention of high blood pressure, it is clearly of more recent origin. This evidence of continuing heart deterioration makes it unlikely that his present heart block will be temporary, as it was the last time. Nevertheless his heart's natural conductivity could return, and vanish, and return again over the following months. The cardiologists decide to fit a "demand" pacemaker that monitors its wearer's own heart and delivers a stimulus only if the natural conductivity fails. The cardiac unit at Boole's is too small to hold stocks of this special device, though it can be on hand within 12 hours. To see Van L. through the night they push a solid, conductive catheter up a vein into his right ventricle and couple it to an external pacemaker. With his heart beating normally he returns to full consciousness. And because his data was on file at center, the first thing he hears is that not only has his wife been told of his accident, she is actually waiting to see him.

Such dispatch—in both the welfare and the medical problems posed by his admission—is characteristic of the benefits that follow the automation of a hospital's data-handling processes, especially when it takes in all the other hospitals in the area. Here was a man admitted unconscious and not far from death; in his pocket, a single name that might or might not have been his. Unknown to his doctors he has a coronary history and has been treated for it in a nearby hospital. In precomputer days they would have chanced giving him the isopropylnorepinephrine, and in his drowsy and uncooperative semiconsciousness, they, might have pried some details out of him. It could have taken days to get all his records over from the other hospital. And his wife could have spent a very worried evening wondering where he was. But because they got all the data they needed in less than an hour, the doctors could act quickly and correctly.

Even so, this represents a small fraction of the benefits the system can bring. To grasp their full scope we must shift our focus away from the individual patient and see how the various departments and services at Boole's are all meshed into the data network. Let us do this by following a sample of blood from Van Leeuwenhoek down to the biochemistry laboratory.

When he wakes the following morning, his first visitor is a records clerk. The clerk has many of Van Leeuwenhoek's details from the stored data—full name, address, date of birth, next of kin, etc. Van Leeuwenhoek checks them while the clerk gets

Northfleet Hospital Group
BOOLE'S MEMORIAL HOSPITAL

registration	230847
sex	M
ward	CAR
surname	VAN LEEUWENHOEK
marital status	MARRIED
first forename	VIVIAN
second forename	
maiden name	
previous surname	
date of birth	29:02:32
age	37
religion	
date of admission	01:03:69
accident location	0
consultant	0512 PROF. MICHAELS
category	C
source	A
patient's address	619 MAIN STREET NORTHFLEET LONDON N8
occupation	Production Manager
next of kin and address	(Mrs) Dorothy V.L. 619 Main Street

In the standard admissions form at Boole's (shown above) the first 18 entries are done on a typewriter linked to a card-punching machine; the rest are filled by hand. The typewritten entries can be duplicated (by the spirit duplication process) onto other humanly readable documents. The card puncher produces the cards 2A and 3A illustrated on the next page.

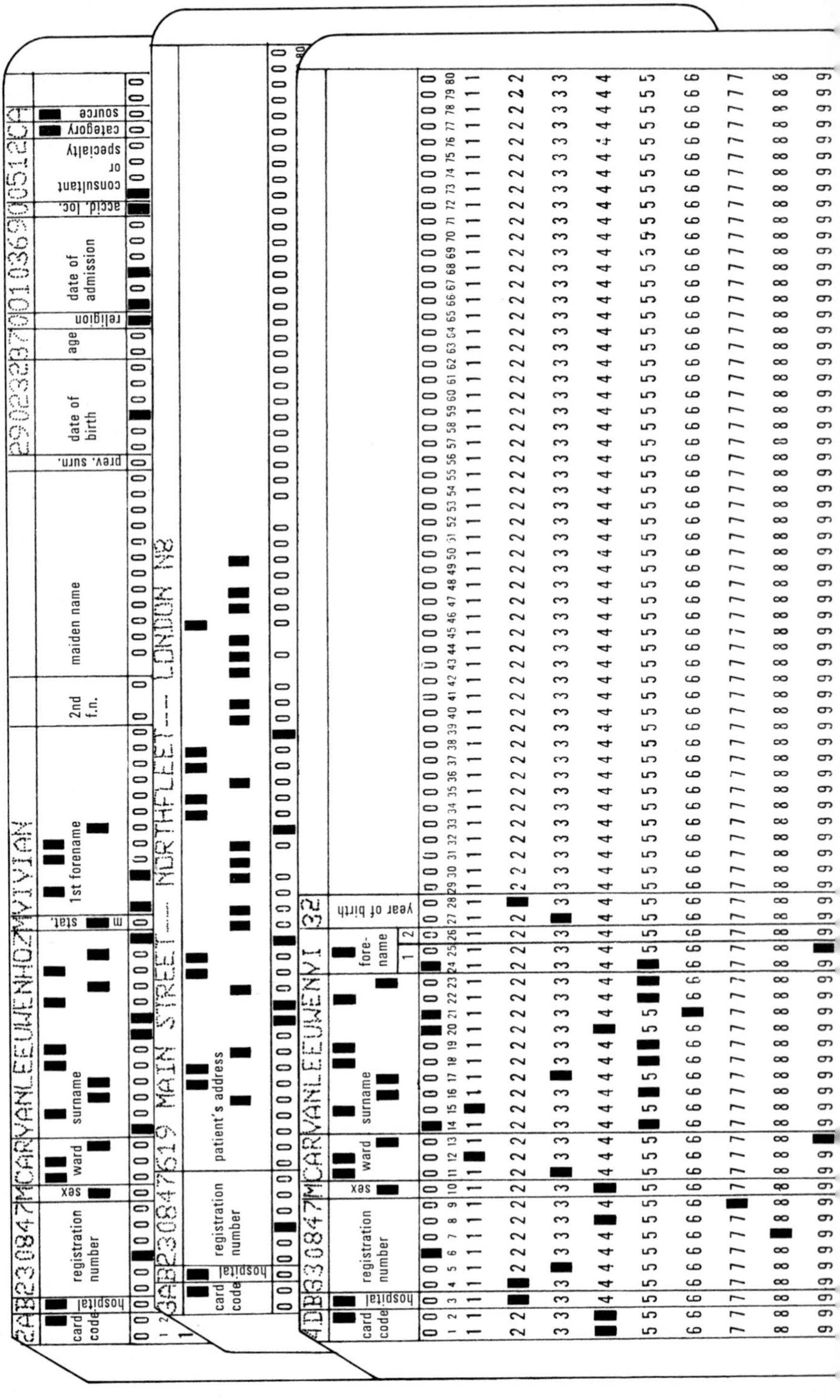
card code
hospital
registration number
sex
ward
surname
stat.
1st forename
2nd f.n.
maiden name
prev. surn.
date of birth
age
religion
date of admission
accid. loc.
consultant or specialty
category
source
patient's address
fore-name
year of birth

other details from the ward sister. Both sets of details are combined in a master of the kind shown on page 129. The typed details in the right-hand column can be duplicated down the margin of other documents by a spirit-duplication system. The typewriter itself is coupled through local 1 to a card punch, which turns out the two master cards shown partly obscured opposite. The card that obscures them, the short master, is automatically produced immediately after the two masters; it is the key to the entire system. It is the medium through which the people in the hospital tell the computer what is happening.

Every interdepartmental transaction is mediated by cards whose first 28 fields are identical with those on the short master. These identify, in order: the card (2 fields), hospital (1), registration number (6), ward (3), sex (1), surname (10—note the further cut from 13 fields on the full master), first two letters of first forename and initial letter of second name (3), and last two figures of year of birth (2), It is important to realize that these cards are not mere *records* of transactions, they are the actual *medium*. Consider the biochemical request cards that we are taking as an example of all such transactions.

Six such cards are automatically generated for each patient on admission. The fifth is especially coded with an instruction to generate a further 6. The 6 cards, together with a lot of other cards for other purposes, are placed in the patient's folder, which holds all his clinical notes.

The day after Van Leeuwenhoek's admission the cardiologists want to see whether he has had a recent coronary attack; because of the previous attacks the EKG is equivocal on this point. If he has had a recent attack, part of his heart will be dying and its cells releasing enzymes (known to physiologists as SGOT, SGPT, and LDH) into his blood. When the doctor has withdrawn a 10-ml sample of blood, all the nurse has to do is to mark the first biochemical card in the way shown on page 132, and then send it down with the sample.

Punch cards (shown opposite) produced at admission are the basis of the hospital's man-machine communications system. Cards 2A and 3A are automatically produced as explained on this page. Card 4D is then generated by the computer, which is programmed to cut the surname to 10 fields, the first forename to 2, the second to 1, and to add the year of birth. Card 4D is used as a master for six 5R cards—and, in fact, for all other interdepartmental cards.

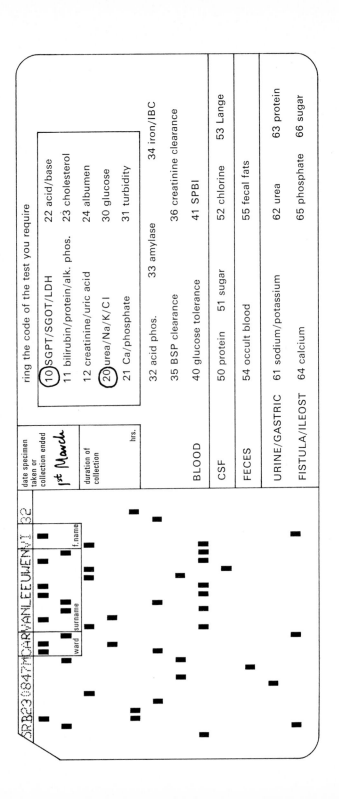

387212	M	WILKINSON	PEW	11.010	010369	
239175	F	JENKINS	MA	20.056	010369	
239175	F	JENKINS	MA	22.006	010369	
239175	F	JENKINS	MA	34.002	010369	
795218	F	GAN	SAT	23.017	010369	
795218	F	GAN	SAT	31.009	010369	
846256	M	WOOD	DAA	20 057	010369	
105742	M	OHALLORAN	FER	20.058	010369	
105742	M	OHALLORAN	FER	30.047	010369	
230847	M	VANLEEUWEN	VI	10.017	010369	
230847	M	VANLEEUWEN	VI	20.059	010369	
449271	F	HODGES	KAC	20.060	010369	
449271	F	HODGES	KAC	00.000	010369	EX
736295	M	TEMPLE	BRS	20.061	010369	

Daysheet (above), showing all tests requested, and a jobsheet (below) for each specific test, are produced by local 2 for internal biochemical laboratory use. These illustrations assume that tests for Van Leeuwenhoek's blood electrolytes and urea were done and entered manually.

239175	CAR	JENKINS	MA	20	056	010369
846256	OPA	WOOD	DAA	20	057	010369
105742	WA2	OHALLORAN	FER	20	058	010369
230847	CAR	VANLEEUWEN	VI	20	059	010369
449271	GYO	HODGES	KAC	20	060	010369
736295	W3B	TEMPLE	BRS	20	061	010369

It so happens that the SGOT/SGPT/LDH determinations are done on a Multichannel machine. This automatically does all the tests whose codes are in the vertical box (codes 10 to 31), so that all the results for those tests will be returned to the ward. (The tests are still listed separately on the card because there are times when they are done manually—on weekends and in emergencies, for instance.) The card acts as input for the biochemistry laboratory's own computer, local 2. For tests on the Multi-channel, local 2 punches the patient's number on the vial that holds the blood (see photograph on page 65). For manual tests, such as the emergency electrolyte determination that was done on Van Leeuwenhoek's blood within an hour of his arrival, local 2 generates a daysheet for all tests and a jobsheet for each specific test (see illustrations above). The manual results are

Opposite: biochemical request card (5R) contains entries of all common tests. All the nurse or doctor has to do is to ring the test required and add the date. The reverse of the card has space for special tests and instructions, diagnosis, and consultant's name or signature. The card is input for local 2.

BIOCHEMICAL TEST RESULTS

card code	hospital	registration number	sex	ward	surname	fore-name 1 2	year of birth	test spec.	spec. recd. D M D	specimen taken D M Y	comment	other

SGPT	SGOT	LDH	bili.	prot.	alk. phos.	serum creat.	uric acid
urea	Na	K	Cl	Ca	phos.	pH	HCO₃	chol.	alb.
sugar	turb.	acid phos.	amyl.	iron	IBC	min. %	min. %	%	creat. clear.
time	sug.	time	sug.	time	sug.	time	sug.	SPBi
prot.	sugar	Cl	Lange	OB	fat
volume	Na	K	urea	prot.	Ca	PO₄	sugar

Opposite: the results card generated from manually entered tests in the completed jobsheets. Such cards, fed into local 2, enable the computer to correct all results for bias and deviation before printing them out for use back in the ward.

Part of the standard form for taking cardiac histories is shown below. Instead of writing out lengthy sentences, the doctor fills boxes on the form.
A punch-card operator turns these entries into cards, on which the data are held in condensed form. Data are similarly condensed in the computer store.
Items that cannot easily be coded (such as associated symptoms and the doctor's remarks) are most economically entered as plain-language sentences.

CURRENT SYMPTOMS

Presenting symptoms

Duration   years   weeks
[ ][ ]   [0][6]

1 *Indigestion*
2 *Angina*
3

Frequency

weeks [ ][ ]

4
5

days [ ][ ]

6
7

hours [1][2]

8
9

almost constant [ ]

10

Pattern

Patient's own words

Gripping

localized   ☒
or
radiating to
jaw   arm   back   epigastrium
☐   ☐   ☐   ☐

Onset		Relief		Recent change in			
eating	☒	rest	☒	severity			☐
exercize	☐	drugs	☐	frequency			☒

Recent change in
weeks   days   hours   almost constant
[ ][ ]   [ ][ ]   [ ][ ]   ☒

		avoidance of		Associated symptoms	
emotion	☐	exercize	☐	indigestion	☐
night	☒	cold	☐	flatulence	
				doom feeling	

Days off work [ ][8]

Remarks *I don't think the pain after fatty meals is significant here*

other (specify) *Pain after fatty meals*

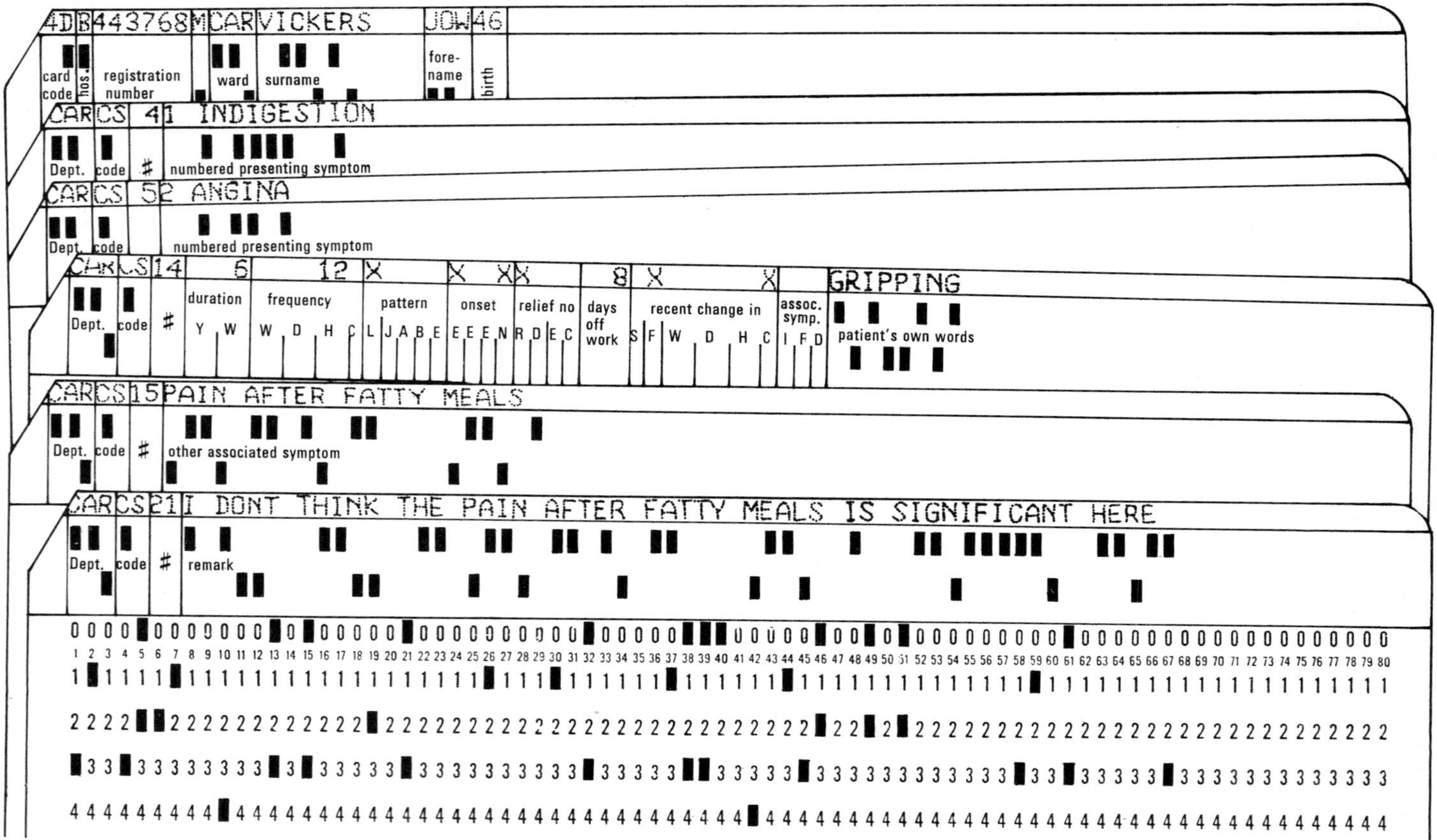

ADB443768M CARVICKERS JOHN 46

| card code | * sou | registration number | ward | surname | fore-name | birth |

CARCS 41 INDIGESTION
Dept. code | # | numbered presenting symptom

CARCS 52 ANGINA
Dept. code | # | numbered presenting symptom

CARCS14 5 12 X X 8 X 8 X X

| duration | frequency | pattern | onset | relief no | days off work | recent change in symp. | assoc. symp. |
| Y W | W D H | J A B E F L | E E E | E N R D E C | | S F W D H C | I F D |

CARCS15 PAIN AFTER FATTY MEALS
Dept. code | # | other associated symptom

GRIPPING
patient's own words

CARCS21 I DONT THINK THE PAIN AFTER FATTY MEALS IS SIGNIFICANT HERE
Dept. code | # | remark

```
MORISON, WHO WAS THE REFERRING DOCTOR.

PRESENTING SYMPTOMS:

INDIGESTION
ANGINA


VICKERS WAS FIT UNTIL 6 WKS AGO WHEN HE FELT A ''GRIPPING''
LOCALIZED CHEST PAIN AT NIGHT AFTER EATING. INITIAL
FREQUENCY WAS EVERY 12 HRS RECENTLY INCREASING TO ALMOST
CONTINUOUS BUT WITHOUT RECENT CHANGE IN SEVERITY. HIS
PAIN IS RELIEVED BY REST. HE HAS BEEN OFF WORK FOR THE LAST
8 DAYS. HE HAS PAIN AFTER FATTY MEALS. (IDONT THINK THE
PAIN AFTER FATTY MEALS IS SIGNIFICANT HERE.)

CHEST SOUNDS.
```

*A special program enables the computer to turn, for instance, the entries
"VICKERS" in fields 14–20 of card 4D and "6" in field 11 of card CARCS 14
(shown opposite) into the statement VICKERS WAS FIT UNTIL 6 WKS AGO.
The program then goes on to turn all other such entries into a plain-language
output as shown above.*

transferred from the jobsheets onto punch cards (see illustration
on page 134), which are then read into local 2 store. The Multichannel returns the results automatically to local 2. Both sets
are stored until the day's end, unless the card was marked
"urgently needed."

Before printing out the results, local 2 runs a number of statistical tests aimed at detecting observer bias, or a drift in values.
If drift or bias is detected, the results are corrected before local
2 prints them out. In precomputer days the calculations were so
lengthy that corrections were unavailable until the following
day—by which time the doctors up in the wards might already
have acted on faulty information. Once again, you see, the computer's ability to store and retrieve, to collate, and to analyze
statistically brings benefits that, though theoretically available
without computers, are in practice unobtainable.

Another use of the cards is seen in the illustrations on pages
135 to 137, showing how part of a patient's cardiac history is
coded for storage; the final illustration shows how the codes
convert back into plain language. Enough has been said of
punch cards to make this example self-explanatory.

Computers in Hospital Organization

Having now studied these two very different applications of punch cards we can easily imagine how they are used either to mediate or to record the hospital's business. At Boole's there are 9 categories in which punch cards are so used; they are listed briefly and numbered in the upper part of the chart opposite. The cardiac history, for instance, is part of category 1; the biochemical requisition is in category 3, which also covers X rays, respiratory tests, EKGs, etc; the results are in category 4. At this point one ought to stress that data in these categories existed and was recorded before computers were thought of. The computer has contributed nothing to medicine except speed in handling existing data. But just look at all that follows such a contribution!

Below the categories is a chart of activities made possible first by a computerized analysis of each separate category (1, 2, 3, 4, etc.), then by correlation and comparison of various combinations (1 + 2 + 9, etc.). Most of these activities are not even attempted in hospitals without computers; those that are attempted, such as prediction of ward status and checks on drugs and side effects, are done well by those who have a flair for the work, badly by those who have not. Overall, the results are so patchy as to make comparisons between hospitals, between departments even, impossible. Let us expand briefly, aphoristically even, on a selection from the list. Obviously we have now finished with "Boole's" and are discussing computers and hospitals in a general context. Only those features that exist routinely at the time of writing are discussed in the present tense.

1. Improved correlation of disease with family history. At the moment we know that many diseases and conditions have an inherited component but it is difficult to quantify; when we can quantify we shall be able to reassure some patients and warn others to look for early symptoms.

Improved correlation of symptoms (*intensity, frequency, and duration*) *with diagnosis.* This will enable us to rank symptoms in precise order of significance. Such studies will also be basic to any future computer-diagnosis program.

2. Hospital and neighborhood profiles. Helps planners to quantify

1	2	3	4	5
Family history, clinical data, & diagnosis	Census-type records	Transfers between wards	Requisitions for services	Results of tests

6	7	8	9
Therapy, drugs, diet, radiation dosage, etc.	Operations	Daily notes on progress	Discharge or death

1	improved correlation of disease with family history
1+2+9	epidemiological studies identification of at-risk patients
1+3+9	prediction of ward status day by day
1+5	ranges of normal and abnormal findings in relation to diagnosis
1+5+6	check on drugs and side effects check on dosages and main therapeutic effects
1+5+6+8	correlation between medical success & age/sex/drug/ physician/diet/etc forecast of drug usage
1+5+7+8	correlation between surgical success and age/sex/surgeon/ technique/etc
1+6+7	prediction of patient's demand on facilities
1+9	morbidity statistics
2	hospital and neighborhood profiles
3	daily lists update
3+4+6	correlation between delays and breakdowns or bottlenecks
4	use of facilities prediction of trends in use
5	quality of control of test results in real time instant check on reading bias by technicians
6	therapeutic profiles by hospital/department/ward/doctor/etc
6+7+9	follow-up of iatrogenic risks
7	surgical profiles by hospital/department/ward/surgeon/etc
8	location of weaknesses in hospital/diet/regime/etc
9	Social Security statistics (disablement/need for appliances of chronic therapy/etc)

needs and to assign priorities; essential not just in maintaining and renewing hospital services but in provision, location, etc. of new hospitals and clinics.

3. Daily lists update. Takes a lot of work off the ward sister's hands.

4. Use of facilities. Enables proper queues and appointments systems to be maintained.

Prediction of trends of use. Analysis of imminent admissions from outpatients' waiting list helps accurate forecasting.

5. Quality control of test results in real time, and *instant check on reading bias by technicians.* We saw how this happened in the clinical biochemistry laboratory. It helps reduce the uncertainty that attended many precomputer readings.

6. Therapeutic profiles by hospital/department/ward/doctor/etc. Doctors are not going to like this one, for it cuts through a number of cherished delusions they have about themselves. Administrators will not be too happy, either, because this will pinpoint inadequacies that they can at present claim are characteristic of the whole of medicine. There will be a strict ban on publication of results under this section—but the doctors will break the ban if results are good; if they are bad, the disgruntled will leak them. Within a decade or two, however, doctors will learn to accept that their performance is continuously measured, both quantitatively and qualitatively—and rightly so.

7. Surgical profiles by hospital/department/ward/surgeon/etc. As for 6 above. At the moment most surgical departments "process" their success rates to "conform with the optima of prevailing norms." Computers won't make consistent exaggerations without very complex programming.

8. Location of weaknesses in hospital. These might be related to diet, wound-infection rates, quality of nursing staff, etc.

9. Social Security statistics. These would help plan aftercare facilities, locate the demand for chronic out-patient therapy, and cut down delays in providing limbs and other appliances.

1 + 2 + 9. Epidemiological studies. These studies have been done on pilot scale with computers. When they are permanent we shall learn a great deal about the relationship between (on the one hand) disease, abnormality, and accident, and (on the other) home environment, education, income, job, habits, diet, etc.

Identification of at-risk patients. We may expect the epidemiological studies to reveal and quantify many risks that are now either concealed or too vaguely known to justify any action. We shall then be able to mass-survey those who undergo such risks and possibly prevent diseases, or at least catch them early.

1 + 3 + 9. Prediction of ward status day by day. This facility improves bed occupancy and produces lower costs per patient per day.

1 + 5. Ranges of normal and abnormal findings in relation to diagnosis. Our need for greater precision in defining "normal" was covered at length in Chapter 3.

1 + 5 + 6. Check on drugs and side effects. This will be of great value in clinical trials of new drugs, and will also reveal low-probability side effects of established drugs.

Check on dosages and main therapeutic effects. At the moment we relate dosages mostly to body weight. We underplay such other factors as obesity, temperature, endocrine activity, bowel, liver, kidney function, previous drug history—because the mathematics involved cannot be done at the bedside. If the computer can do it for us, we might considerably refine our idea of the "correct dosage." (Also we might, at last, discover the limits of homeopathic medicine; the subject is too complex to expand here, but if you are interested, you will find a fair summary in Martin Gardner's *Fads and Fallacies in the Name of Science,* Dover (New York, 1957).

1 + 5 + 6 + 8. Correlation between medical success and age/sex/ drug/physician/etc. This is a more detailed breakdown of data obtainable under 6 alone. For comments, see 6 above.

1 + 5 + 7 + 8. Correlation between surgical success and age/sex/ drug/surgeon/etc. A more detailed breakdown of data obtainable under 7 alone. For comments, see 7 above.

1 + 6 + 7. Prediction of patient's demand on facilities. Essential to economic and efficient deployment of services and staff.

1 + 9. Morbidity statistics. These will be continually available— instead of two years behind, as now.

3 + 4 + 6. Delays, breakdown, bottlenecks. Today these are often noticed too late, so that their effects reverberate back and forth through the system. Early automatic detection and counteraction will greatly ease hospital administration.

6 + 7 + 9. Follow-up of iatrogenic risks. As Dr. James Crooks of the University of Aberdeen, Scotland, has pointed out, iatrogenic disease (disease that arises directly out of therapy) is a growing problem in advanced societies. For instance, the complications that follow gastric surgery, usually to relieve a peptic ulcer, include anemia and bone disease. Although this link is well known Crooks has shown that over 30 per cent of postgastrectomy patients are likely to have untreated anemia and that 10 per cent (who are not necessarily among the anemics) will develop bone disease many years after surgery. He also cites the incidence of thyroid deficiency after the irradiation of diseased thyroid glands—the peak incidence coming eight years after treatment. The problem is severe among older patients because the symptoms can easily be taken for the onset of senility: hoarseness, deafness, intolerance of cold, constipation, sensations of numbness and tingling, dry skin, and so on.

In both cases it is the late onset of the iatrogenic disease and its possible confusion with natural ageing that sharpens the problem. And, as Crooks points out, there are many other patients similarly placed: all cases of gastric surgery, all who are on chronic drug therapy, and all patients undergoing lifelong replacement therapy for chronic anemia, hormone, and nutritional deficiencies. I believe we *owe* it to these patients to minimize the iatrogenic risks we ask them to face; and the computer offers the cheapest and most effective way of controlling the follow up. Each year after the treatment the computer sends a questionnaire to the patient, who takes it to his doctor to be completed and returned. The computer calls in those patients whose questionnaires show positive signs of the iatrogenic condition.

1 + 5 + 6 + 7 + 8. Doctor-computer conversations at cathode-ray tube terminal with light pen. The photograph opposite shows a doctor using such a facility, which is already standard equipment in aircraft and car design studios and architects' and engineering offices. An engineer, for instance, can draw a bridge structure on the CRT (cathode-ray tube) display and the computer will work out stresses and strains under varying conditions of load, crosswind, temperature, and seismic stress. An architect can draw a room plan and then vary the positions and sizes of the windows until he gets, say, optimum lighting for minimum cost. In all such applications the user is asking the computer, "What if . . . ?"—"What if I took out this cross brace? . . . moved this window? . . . made it smaller?" and so on. And he is getting answers without the cost and delay of building actual structures or models. The analogue in medicine would be for the doctor to ask, "What if I changed the dosage to such and such while reducing the diet in this or that way?" and so on. If he could get reliable answers he could optimize his therapy without involving the patient in the preliminary hunt for the optimum.

The light pen held by this doctor at the Mayo Clinic provides a means of instant communication with the computer, which displays data on the screen. If the doctor wants to record, or write, or erase any of the data so displayed, he points the light pen at the entry and presses the appropriate key. A keyboard beside the terminal enables undisplayed data to be put in.

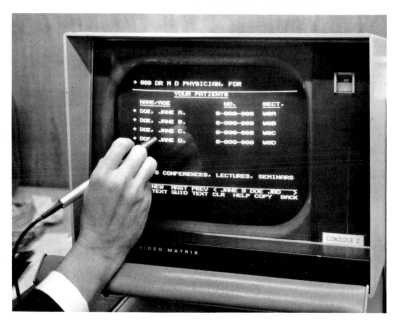

```
 000  DR  M  D  PHYSICIAN,  FOR

               YOUR PATIENTS

    NAME                NO           SECT
 ●  DOE, JANE A.        0-000-000    WBA
    DOE, JANE B.        0-000-000    WBB
    DOE, JANE C.        0-000-000    WBC
    DOE, JANE D.        0-000-000    WBD




       S  CONFERENCES.  LECTURES.  SEMINARS

       NEW    MAST   PREV    JANE  A   DOE  JAD
 ERR   TEXT   GUID   TEXT    CLR   HELP  COPY BACK
```

1 Doctor identifies himself to computer, which prints his patient list.

```
 000  DR  M  D  PHYSICIAN  FOR  JANE  A  DOE
 AT 13:33, 10/20/67
              M A S T E R      G U I D E

 PHYSICIAN ENTRY

    GENERAL INFORMATION
    FAMILY HISTORY
    SOCIAL HISTORY
    PAST HISTORY
    INVENTORY BY SYSTEMS

 ●  PHYSICAL EXAM

    SYMPTOMS BY SPECIALITY
    SYMPTOMS BY DIAGNOSIS
    SYMPTOMS BY ALPHABETIC LISTING



       NEW    MAST   PREV    JANE  A   DOE  JAD
 ERR   TEXT   GUID   TEXT    CLR   HELP  COPY BACK
```

2a Computer records time/date; doctor indicates next entry category . . .

```
    PHYSICAL EXAM
    AT 13:33, 10/20/67
              PHYSICAL GUIDE

 NORM    NO EXAM      VITAL SIGNS
 NORM    NO EXAM      GEN OBSERVATIONS
 NORM    NO EXAM      SCALP
 NORM    NO EXAM      SKIN
 NORM    NO EXAM      EARS
 NORM    NO EXAM      EYES
 NORM    NO EXAM      NOSE
 NORM    NO EXAM      ORAL CAVITY-THROAT
 NORM    NO EXAM      SALIVARY GLANDS
 NORM    NO EXAM      LYMPH NODES
 NORM    NO EXAM      THYROID
 NORM    NO EXAM      BREASTS
 NORM    NO EXAM      PERIPHERAL VESSELS
 NORM    NO EXAM   ●  HEART

                      GUIDE CONT
                      MASTER GUIDE
       NEW    MAST   PREV    JANE  A   DOE  JAD
 ERR   TEXT   GUID   TEXT    CLR   HELP  COPY BACK
```

2b Doctor selects appropriate item from general physical guide.

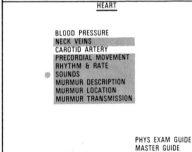

```
    PHYSICAL EXAM
    HEART
                            HEART

        BLOOD PRESSURE
        NECK VEINS
        CAROTID ARTERY
        PRECORDIAL MOVEMENT
        RHYTHM & RATE
     ●  SOUNDS
        MURMUR DESCRIPTION
        MURMUR LOCATION
        MURMUR TRANSMISSION




                           PHYS EXAM GUIDE
                           MASTER GUIDE
       NEW    MAST   PREV    JANE  A   DOE  JAD
 ERR   TEXT   GUID   TEXT    CLR   HELP  COPY BACK
```

3b Each above category can generate a further matrix, for example . . .

```
    HEART
    SOUNDS
                      HEART SOUNDS

 S1          NORMAL          ACCENTUATED GRADE
 S2   AORT   LOUD               1    2    3    4
      PULM   ABSENT
 S3          PRESENT
 S4          FIXED                    AND
             PARADOXICAL

                     EARLY     TRANSIENT
 EJECTION SOUND      MID       PROBABLE
 SYSTOLIC CLICK      SYST      QUESTIONABLE
 OPENING SNAP        DIAST
 PERICARDIAL RUB     SHORT
 S2-O/S INTERVAL     MEDIUM
                     LONG
                  ●  MURMURS DESC
                     HEART EXAM GUIDE
                     PHYS EXAM GUIDE
                     MASTER GUIDE
       NEW    MAST   PREV    JANE  A   DOE  JAD
 ERR   TEXT   GUID   TEXT    CLR   HELP  COPY BACK
```

4b . . . heart sounds (among which the doctor chooses)

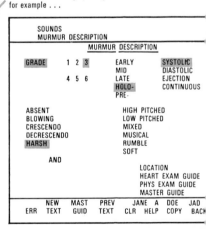

```
    SOUNDS
    MURMUR DESCRIPTION
                    MURMUR DESCRIPTION

 GRADE    1  2  3        EARLY      SYSTOLIC
                        MID        DIASTOLIC
          4  5  6        LATE       EJECTION
                        HOLO-      CONTINUOUS
                        PRE-

 ABSENT                 HIGH PITCHED
 BLOWING                LOW PITCHED
 CRESCENDO              MIXED
 DECRESCENDO            MUSICAL
 HARSH                  RUMBLE
                        SOFT
     AND
                        LOCATION
                        HEART EXAM GUIDE
                        PHYS EXAM GUIDE
                        MASTER GUIDE
       NEW    MAST   PREV    JANE  A   DOE  JAD
 ERR   TEXT   GUID   TEXT    CLR   HELP  COPY BACK
```

5b . . . murmur description, from which the doctor also selects entries.

```
HYSICAL EXAM:
HISTORY:
         CARDIOVASC. SYMPTOM GUIDE

CRAL COLOR CHG        FEVER
NGINA                HEADACHE
HEST PAIN            HEMOPTYSIS
LAUDICATION          HYPERTENSION
LUBBING              HYPERVEN SYNDROME
UTANEOUS ULCER       PALPITATION
YANOSIS              PARESTHESIA
EAFNESS              PREVIOUS C/V DZ:
IPLOPIA              PREVIOUS THERAPY
YSPNEA               SYNCOPE
DEMA                 T.I.A.
XTREMITY PAIN        VERTIGO
ATIGUE               VISION
                     WEAKNESS-MUSCLE

                     SPECIALITY GUIDE
                     MASTER GUIDE
      NEW    MAST    PREV    JANE A DOE  JAD
RR   TEXT   GUID    TEXT   CLR HELP COPY BACK
```

and specific area within that category: chest pain. ⟶

*The diagrams on these pages show
how a doctor can enter details of case
history (a sequence) and results of a
physical examination (b sequence) in
the patient's record simply by
selecting items from prepared
matrixes that cover most
contingencies; rare entries can be
entered by means of the keyboard.
Entries shown in gray figure in the
final assembled message (whose
other entries are similarly arrived at).
Gray dots indicate entries that gain
access to the next matrix here
illustrated.*

```
HISTORY
   CHEST PAIN
                    CHEST PAIN GUIDE

        ONSET
        SEVERITY
        FREQUENCY
        DURATION
        DISABILITY
        COURSE
        LOCATION
        REFERRAL AREAS
    ●   DESCRIPTION
        RELIEF
        AGGRAVATIONS
        ASSOCIATED CONDITIONS

                        SYMPTOM GUIDE
                        CHIEF COMPLAINT
                        MASTER GUIDE
      NEW    MAST    PREV    JANE A DOE  JAD
ERR  TEXT   GUID    TEXT   CLR HELP COPY BACK
```

4a Each above category can generate a further matrix,
for example . . .

```
CHEST PAIN
   DESCRIPTION
            CHEST PAIN DESCRIPTION

MODIFIERS                DESCRIBED AS
DULL            ACHING          PRESSURE
SHARP           BORING          PRICKLING
INTERMITTENT    BURNING         PULLING
                CHOKING         SHOOTING
                CONSTRICTING    STABBING
        AND     CRUSHING        STICKING
                FULLNESS        TEARING
                HEAVINESS       THROBBING
                KNIFELIKE       TIGHTNESS

                    ADVANCE
                    DESC GUIDE
                    SYMPTOM GUIDE
                    CHIEF COMPLAINT
                    MASTER GUIDE
      NEW    MAST    PREV    JANE A DOE  JAD
ERR  TEXT   GUID    TEXT   CLR HELP COPY BACK
```

5a . . . chest pain description— in this case "constricting
and crushing."

```
      PAGE MODE—ASSEMBLED MESSAGE

000  DR M D PHYSICIAN, FOR JANE A DOE ↵
     AT 13:39, 10/20/67
HYSICAL EXAM:
   HEART:
   NECK VEINS: ESTIMATED PRESSURE 3 CM
   ABOVE STERNAL NOTCH
   PRECORDIAL MOVEMENT LT VENT LIFT
   LOCALIZED TO 5 I C S AT M C L
   RYTHM & RATE: FREQUENT PREMATURE BEATS
   HEART SOUNDS: AORT S2 ABSENT
   MURMUR DESCRIPTION: GRADE 3 HARSH
   HOLO- SYSTOLIC
   MURMUR LOCATION: APEX &, BEST HEARD
   SUPINE POSITION
   TRANSMISSION AXILLA

                 PREV      JANE A DOE JAD
ETURN           TEXT   ASSEMBLE COPY ENTER
```

tes under 6a also apply here. Correlation of symptoms
gns with final diagnosis will help computer gain
rience" at diagnosis.

```
      PAGE MODE—ASSEMBLED MESSAGE

000  DR M D PHYSICIAN, FOR JANE A DOE
     AT 13:39, 10/20/67
HISTORY
   CHEST PAIN:.
   ONSET: ABRUPT ABOUT 2 YRS AGO
   SEVERITY: MILD AT ONSET AND SEVERE
   PAST 4 MOS:
   FREQUENCY: EPISODICALLY ABOUT EVERY
   2 WKS & LAST OCCURRED 2 DAYS AGO.
   DURATION: USUALLY 2-4 MIN.
   DISABILITY: INCAPACITATING PAST 24
   HRS.
   LOCATION: SUBSTERNAL AREA.
   REFERRAL AREAS: LEFT UPPER ARM &
   JAW
   DESCRIPTION: CONSTRICTING & CRUSHING
   RELIEF: DEFINITELY NITROGLYCERINE &
   OCCASIONALLY ALCOHOL

                 PREV      JANE A DOE JAD
RETURN          TEXT   ASSEMBLE COPY ENTER
```

6a Entries from previous matrixes are assembled to make
page from complete history. Doctor can revise any entry and
ask for a printout.

It will be a long time before computers can be used in this way in medicine: the variables of human response are too complex, and their interdependence too obscure (as yet), for us to write any useful program to relate them. But, as the photograph shows, the same CRT can be used in a humbler role as a presenter and acquirer of data, a time-saving interface between the doctor and the hospital computer system. The system illustrated is at the Mayo Clinic, Rochester, Minnesota and is used for acquisition of patient data for the medical record, for ordering tests, and for assisting the doctor in planning a diagnostic sequence.

Diagrams on pages 144 and 145 (retyped from actual CRT displays for clarity) show how part of "Jane Doe's" cardiac history might be entered. As you see, the doctor is faced with a sequence of possible entries, each of which is backed by a list of subentries, each item in which is further backed up—and so on until all but the rarest possibilities are exhausted. Each such list, or *matrix*, is called up by pointing the light pen at the appropriate entry and pressing a button that calls up the matrix of that entry's subentries. In the present system the doctor types nothing except rare conditions, or such qualifications as *about, definitely, occasionally, approximately*, and so on. Other entries are automatically incorporated into the history when the doctor points the light pen at them and presses the appropriate button. Parts of two sequences are shown: one leads to a record of Jane Doe's history, the other to a record of her physical examination. The advantages of such a system are: the resulting records are to a standard format; they are far more complete than traditional records; they are legible (no mean benefit); they are instantly retrievable—either in printed form or on CRT display; and they are entered instantaneously instead of the doctor having to take notes, dictate to a secretary, and get them typed at length. Suitably programmed, the computer can hoard its "experience" (actually, the experience of all the doctors who use it) and begin to calculate the probabilities that any given symptom, sign, or test result will correlate with any given disease. In time this will become a valuable aid to diagnosis itself. It will certainly help to train doctors, whether they are beginners or have fallen behind the times; an experienced computer could respectfully point out to

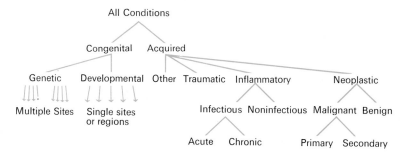

A diagnostic sieve is used by doctors, consciously or unconsciously, while diagnosing patients. A typical example is the one I use, shown above. Often the condition is obvious enough to start partway down (a gunshot wound, for instance, is obviously traumatic). As described in the text, my path through this tree involves leaps of insight or observation of a kind difficult to program. At the most detailed level shown here, the current view is turning into a provisional diagnosis. It is at this level that diagnostic machines and computers can help.

a doctor that he has associated a given set of signs or symptoms with a certain diagnosis and that such an association has never before been made—would he like to recheck? Of course, the doctor may be quite right, but it would be valuable to have this double check built into the system.

With the Mayo facility similar matrixes are displayed to a doctor who wants to order a test on a patient. Again the advantages are of speed, standardization of format, and a reduction in secretarial and paper work. There is the added advantage of flexibility, for whereas in most hospitals the types of forms on which a doctor can order, say, biochemical tests is limited, for obvious administrative reasons, the computer and CRT can generate order forms for any number of purposes. For instance, in the course of a day a doctor may want to order biochemical tests for a whole variety of purposes: to test organ function (liver, thyroid), to determine a given constituent (fat, say, which includes tests for at least six substances in the plasma), to check on therapy, or to help in diagnosis. In an ideal hospital (which I define as a place run solely for patients and those who treat them) there would be separate order forms for each purpose. The CRT

PLEASE TELL ME ABOUT THE PATIENT

The patient with me here is 23 years old

PLEASE CONTINUE

He shows no evidence of cyanosis

OK PLEASE GO ON

There is no indication of the squatting symptom

ALL RIGHT. GO ON PLEASE

I'm afraid that's all I know about him at present

CHECK THE HILAR VESSELS. ARE THEY INCREASED OR DECREASED

They are increased

I SEE
LOOK FOR A LEFT SECOND SYSTOLIC MURMUR

First tell me what the three most probable diseases are at this time

 2 WITH PROBABILITY 74
18 WITH PROBABILITY 7
30 WITH PROBABILITY 3
PLEASE CONTINUE
LOOK FOR A LEFT SECOND SYSTOLIC MURMUR

What is the medical name of disease 2

ATRIAL SEPTAL DEFECT
OK PLEASE GO ON
LOOK FOR A LEFT SECOND SYSTOLIC MURMUR

and the name of disease 18 is

PATENT DUCTUS ARTERIOSUS
ALL RIGHT. GO ON PLEASE
LOOK FOR A LEFT SECOND SYSTOLIC MURMUR

He has a left second systolic murmur

ALL RIGHT
IS THE AXIS IN THE ECG RIGHT, LEFT, OR NORMAL

It is a right axis

OK
I RECOMMEND A DIAGNOSIS OF DISEASE 2

What is your current view of the problem

MY CURRENT VIEW IS
DISEASE PROBABILITY

| 2 | 93 |
| 4 | 2 |

Name disease 4 for me

ATRIAL SEPTAL DEFECT WITH PULMONARY HYPERTENSION

I'm finished with this case. Thank you for your help

I HOPE THAT I HAVE BEEN OF SERVICE. GOODBYE

terminal allows the computer to generate such forms so that the doctor can select, say, a fat test and leave the computer to specify: cholesterol, cholesterol esterase, fatty acids, lipids total, phospholipid, and triglyceride. On the manual order form, which is a compromise among all the various possible forms, "cholesterol" might well be buried among "carb diox., chlorine, creatinine . . ." and "phospholipid" might figure among "PHTSE acid, PHTSE alk, phosphorus, potassium. . . ."

The most interesting use of the Mayo computer system is in the strategic planning of a diagnostic sequence. In examining a patient the doctor starts off with very limited information, too limited to allow diagnosis but sufficient for him to form a current view. As he proceeds, this view is either hardened or modified until the probability that the patient has this or that condition is as high as the doctor, using all his training and experience, can put it; at that moment the current view becomes a diagnosis. The early and most important parts of the process involve large, heuristic, mental leaps that are far beyond the powers of any machine—as yet. The doctor goes through a diagnostic sieve (shown in tree form on page 147) that rapidly reduces the current view from the broadest possibilities to narrower probabilities. Often this process involves associative connections of a kind quite alien to the plodding logic of the computer. I remember as a student seeing a teacher diagnose a lump in a young girl's breast as a bruise, not the tumor or infection everyone else had taken it to be. "It was her two new front teeth gave me the clue," he said, "I thought perhaps someone had hit her about." Who could write a program that could include all such possible changes?

But when the doctor has narrowed his current view down to a provisional diagnosis, he begins to need tests of various kinds—some of them costly in time, staff, and money, and possibly discomforting or even hazardous to the patient. Thus the doctor must become adept at balancing, on the one hand, the probability

In the conversation shown opposite the computer "speaks" in capitals, the doctor in ordinary type. The computer was programmed to choose the most useful (i.e. revealing) test, given certain known facts about the patient. As new facts come in, the strategy changes and the current view hardens into a diagnosis.

that his current view is the correct diagnosis, plus the expected yield (in confirmation or otherwise of his current view) from this or that test, and, on the other hand, the cost to the patient in medical and financial terms and the burden on any staff involved in the test. Notice that the current view determines which tests the doctor orders next, and that the results of the tests, in turn, may modify his current view. The interaction is complex and few doctors would claim that, even routinely, they achieve an optimum path through all possible tests. It is precisely here that the computer can help, for where unknown causes (such as uncertainly diagnosed conditions) have known effects (symptoms, signs, and test results) and where the probability linking any given cause with any particular effect can be stated with fair accuracy, we can use Bayes' theorem to determine the probability of a given diagnosis from the results of the very first test. (In this context Bayes' theorem, propounded as long ago as 1764, states: $P(d_1/R) = \{P(d_1)P(R/d_1)\}/\{\sum P(d_2)P(R/d_2)\}$ where d_1, d_2, $d_3 \ldots d_n$ are a number of mutually exclusive diagnoses one of which must be right, R is an observation or test result, $P(R/d_1)$ is the probability that the result R will occur if diagnosis d_1 is correct, and $P(d_1/R)$ is the probability of diagnosis d_1 after R has been observed—that is, the probability the doctor is seeking to establish. The summation is between $d_2 = 1$ and n.

More important, the computer can use Bayes' theorem to establish which test would do most to increase the diagnostic probability. And the doctor can balance the computer's recommendation against his own knowledge of the risk to the patient (or the cost) and the immediate availability of machines and staff.

The diagram on page 148 shows (retyped for clarity) a doctor-computer dialogue that occurred while diagnostic strategies for congenital heart defects were being evaluated at the Mayo Clinic. To do this the doctor was using records of already diagnosed patients; thus he could respond instantly to the suggestion to "check the hilar vessels" (which carry the lungs' own blood supply), though in a live situation he would have to stop the dialogue and send the patient for an X-ray photo. In this particular program there are 35 congenital heart diseases, producing a total of 57 signs and symptoms. In all, 34 tests were available, of which the program selected, on average, only 6.9 tests per patient to achieve results comparable with those of experts.

Far below Cloud Seven

In writing about computers I have not even felt a temptation to deal with their far-out applications in medicine. Writers who have trodden this path before me have postulated a number of such applications—computer-assisted neurosurgery . . . dialysis . . . drug administration; diagnostic terminals at street corners with access to a national medical grid; public-health sampling points at notorious highway bottlenecks so that the motorist can put his time to good use; and so on. Obviously it is foolhardy to say of any rational human activity that it offers no openings for computers; but it seems to me that in the early 1970s the real excitement of computer applications in medicine lies in the more humdrum fields I have outlined. The data we acquire in the present-day practice of medicine is closer to being an effluent or pollutant of the system than a valuable product. If the computer does little more than reverse the situation, it will, even so, lay the foundation for one of the greatest advances in the entire history of medicine.

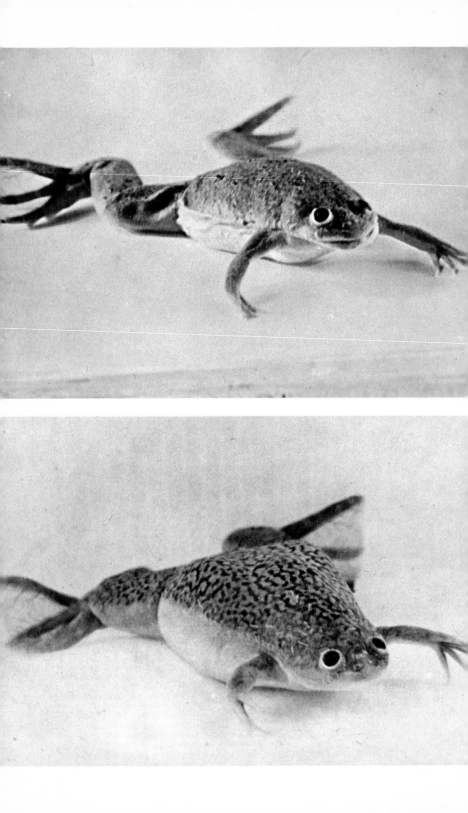

7   Outlook

When the Luftwaffe burned down the British parliament buildings
in World War II it found surprising allies down below—the night
staff of the Houses of Parliament, who refused to let the firecrews
into the building, because only members and servants of parliament had authority to enter there! On the very same night an
incendiary bomb fell into a bonded warehouse, but customs
officers would not let firemen into the premises without the necessary permit. The resulting fire wrecked a sorely needed wharf.

Every age and every country has its own crop of such stories,
which make us heave with weary exasperation. We can be tolerant
of computers that send out bills for $0.00. We do not expect fellow
humans to be quite so punctiliously reflexive. Why, then, are our
expectations so frequently dashed? At the root of all such stories
are systems that require humans to behave like computers:

Q: Has the bearer permit to enter?
A1: Yes—bearer may enter.
A2: No—bearer may not enter.

When such an elementary binary function defines more than 80

The photographs opposite show that all living processes are under chemical
(i.e. genetic) control and illustrate an astounding example of manipulation at
the cellular level. The frog shown at top is a completely normal animal; the one
shown below was produced in the laboratory by replacing the nucleus of an
unfertilized egg cell with the nucleus of a cell taken from the intestine of an
already developed tadpole (see page 164).

per cent of a man's job, and when he does that job for, let's say, 40 years, it is not at all surprising that he behaves with the mulish logic of a computer. Naturally the job is not defined in such bald terms. Its basic algorithm is dressed up in the traditional finery of some service or in-group; and the in-group mentality is fostered by setting up insider-outsider demarcations. Outsiders who want to visit Insideland must apply for permits, state their purposes, and show appropriate gratitude. Those who do not are either spies or poachers.

At this point, scientist-readers may feel a vague twinge of discomfort. Imperceptibly I have moved away from a description of a humble gatekeeper's job to one that fits almost every branch of science—and every branch of medicine. In creative science, success justifies almost any amount of spying and poaching; but in normative science, which is what most scientists practice, either activity is a breach of accepted standards. Of course, we all draw lines around our various areas of work: this is thoracic, that cardiac; this is biochemical, that biophysical; these are neurotic signs, those psychotic; and so on. Such demarcations are useful only as long as we treat them like contour lines—abstract marks on our conceptual map of a given area. They help us to understand how parts of a field are related, but do not prevent us from wandering freely over it. The dangers of the other extreme are obvious—when what should be simple contours sprout pickets of barbed wire and all the other marks of a private preserve. It is in the in-between state—where the fences are genteelly unobtrusive and each specialist's right to "his" preserve is tacitly accepted—that insidious damage can be done.

Nowhere does this argument apply more clearly than in medicine. Our field of study—the human animal, collective and individual—is carved up among several hundred specializations. The divisions are scored ever deeper by our career structure, our methods of funding research, our administrative bodies, and (let us be frank) our very success in each given area of specialization.

In this chapter I shall argue that these divisions ultimately defeat their own purposes, that success achieved by concentrating on one particular area without regard to the whole is quickly subject to a law of diminishing returns, that machines (though not the ones we use today) will play an important part in uniting medicine's fragments, and that if we fail to work toward such unity our goal (a healthy mind in a healthy body in a healthy community) will, like the rainbow's end, recede before us as fast as we pursue it. Peter Ustinov tells a story that reveals the close affinity between specialization and lunacy. A golfer, early in his round, drove a ball clean off the links. When he later got back to the clubhouse he found it in uproar. "What's the matter?" he asked the professional coach. "Have you not heard?" said the pro. "Someone drove off the links and hit a cyclist, who fell in front of a school bus. The bus pulled over to avoid him and overturned down an embankment. Forty children dead." "Good grief!" said the golfer, "I drove that ball. What can I do . . . what can I *do*?" "You could try holding your club a little more like this," said the pro, demonstrating.

There are few specialist doctors who can laugh at this particular story with a completely easy conscience. For most of us our specialities are as important and all-consuming as golf was to that pro. The dunce's cap with which we should have freely crowned the parliamentary watchmen and customs officers of this chapter's first paragraph begins to look and feel uncomfortably like the ceremonial headgear we ourselves wear on formal academic occasions.

This line of thought has been forced on me by my commitment to write this book. From the start I was determined not to compose an extended catalog of medical machinery; instead I set out to describe the fundamental processes on which bio-engineering rests. The determination inevitably focused my thoughts on how research in bio-engineering actually gets done. The conclusions are disturbing.

My work brings me in touch with a fair cross section of the life-involved sciences. My formal job (managing the machines associated with our cardiac surgery unit and recovery wards), for instance, takes me among polymer chemists, metallurgists, and electronic engineers; when mishaps occur I contact forensic scientists, poisons experts, and microbiologists. My research involves me with chemical engineers, filtration scientists, laser physicists, and production engineers. To ensure a good start to the British National Tissue Service (which routes complex homo-graft tissues from donor to recipient hospitals on the basis of tissue compatibility and other factors) I had to meet with im-munologists, radio engineers, systems analysts, and data-pro-cessing specialists. And meetings, lectures, and symposiums allow countless opportunities to participate in the "invisible colleges" that flourish away from the speaker's dais.

This rich web of contact has given me what I now realize to be a fairly privileged view of the sciences that impinge on medi-cine. Yet I am ceaselessly amazed at the amount of knowledge lying around, as it were, in these neighboring sciences—know-ledge vital to medicine, yet unknown to it. Let me give just one example.

Like all cardiac surgery centers we have a number of unex-plained deaths each year. The number is, fortunately, small, but even one unexplained death is too many. We analyzed every possible cause or contributory factor and took a number of evasive actions—including a procedure whereby we set the heart-

These photographs, taken from successive frames of a high-speed cine film, show progressive collapse of a cavitation bubble close to a solid surface. (Time interval between each photograph is 0.5 milliseconds.) The cavity becomes involuted on one side and a jet of water shoots across the bubble at high speed. The great force exerted by such jets is considered to be the cause of cavitation erosion on ships' propellers and on turbines, and has been linked with the polymerization of sugar molecules in blood, described in the text.

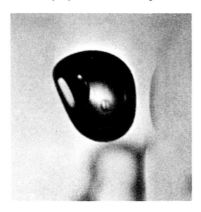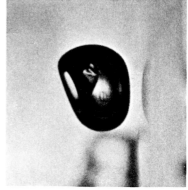

lung machine pumps so that they just failed to occlude as the roller passed over them. We set the pumps in this way to prevent the hemolysis caused when the rough walls that occur in even the finest pump tubing were pressed firmly together by the roller. One day Bob Bass, the aerodynamicist I mentioned in Chapter 5, happened to be watching us set up the pumps in this way, and I explained our reasoning. He was not at all happy with the argument and, after the operation, he demonstrated that under-occlusion (which is bound to occur with this setup) could permit minute streams of turbulent backflow—ideal conditions in which cavitation can occur. (Cavitation is a phenomenon in which tiny vapor bubbles spontaneously form in a liquid when its hydro-static pressure falls below its vapor pressure. The singing of a kettle is caused by the collapse of cavitation bubbles.) Immediate-ly before they collapse, cavitation bubbles develop huge tensions in their walls; and, because they hardly ever collapse symmetric-ally, the forces tend to concentrate on the side collapsing fastest (see the photographs opposite and below). As a result those sides buckle inward and shoot a jet of liquid—called a *Munro jet*—across the bubble. Though the cross-sectional area of the jet is only 0.01 mm², the forces in it are stupendous: 1000 kg/mm²! Such forces, Bob felt, could hemolyze as many red cells as could the overocclusion we were seeking to avoid. Needless to say, none of us medical men had ever heard of Munro jets; but after a day or two's thought it became clear to us that the gigantic

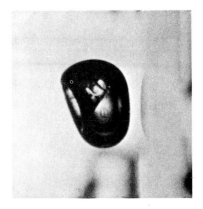
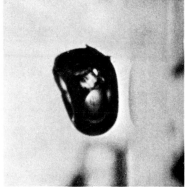

forces they brought to bear on minute areas posed an even more ominous threat than hemolysis: such forces might be great enough to polymerize small sugar molecules into large polysaccharides. The effect of liberating large polysaccharides into the blood was unpredictable, but could only be harmful.

These doubts were raised several months ago. In the meantime we have established that such polymerization does occur and that it is probably related to cavitation; but we have not linked the process with our unexplained deaths. However, the results are merely incidental to my present theme; the main point is that the power of cavitation bubbles to do immense harm has been known for over a century, and one of its most potent mechanisms, the Munro jet, was discovered in the 1940s. It is now quite clear that cavitation must occur in every heart-lung bypass operation and that ways of reducing it must be deliberately sought by designers of future machines. Yet, to judge by the published literature and conversations with colleagues, it had never occurred to anybody to relate the phenomenon to heart-lung machines at all. And—as you have seen—it did not exactly *occur* to us, either. Suppose I had been too preoccupied that day to explain the off-center setup to Bob. Suppose he had been distracted and had listened with only half an ear, or had not come to see us at all. On such slender threads of coincidence does our "discovery" depend!

I could multiply this example several dozen times—as, I am sure, could every medical worker, indeed every scientist. One cannot help wondering how often, how very often, coincidence has worked the other way: depriving us of answers to the many bio-engineering problems that beset us. A few years ago it was commonplace to discern an ever-widening division among the sciences. People envisaged a time when two scientists in closely related fields would hardly understand each other. My experience is precisely the reverse. No matter how obscure and remote-seeming the science with which my work brings me into contact, I find *something* within it that is relevant to the work I or my colleagues are engaged on. Far from growing apart, we have the strongest incentives for uniting; we desperately need a community of action that depends on something more substantial than coincidence.

The classic community of this kind is the Manhattan Project, which led to the first fission bombs. It united just about every known physical and chemical science in one joint effort. If the atom bomb had depended on the haphazard serendipidity we rely on in bio-engineering, the world would still be wondering if Rutherford hadn't been right when he said that the atom would never provide man with a source of power.

What was it that brought together, on the one hand, physicists so abstract that they were practically philosophers and, on the other, high-voltage engineers who tended to scoff at equations that included the square root of −1 in their terms? Clearly it was more than administrative decision, or organization, or money. The nature of the project soon convinced such radically different workers that they belonged on the same team. Above all, though, they were able to relate to one another because the work of men like Einstein, Bohr, Planck, Rutherford, Cockcroft, and Heisenberg had provided a unified conceptual framework for their operation.

It is just such a framework that we lack in bio-engineering—more than money, more than organization, more than administrative backing. The complexity of our subject—life itself, no less—is daunting; there is no hope that some "unified field equations" of physiology will soon pop into some thinker's mind and that the whole field of living matter will suddenly be lit with a single light of crystalline clarity and undreamed-of intensity. Realizing this, implicitly or explicitly, we have concluded that our field has no conceptual unity apart from trivial or obvious statements about life. As a result, designers of, say, therapeutic machines based on ultrasound, kidney machines, and implantable telemetry capsules feel little more in common with each other than with, say, a gas-turbine designer.

Such resignation, I feel, is a little shortsighted. A concept does not have to be universal (like $E=mc^2$) in order to provide a framework of unity in our field. But it must be fundamental enough to relate, for instance, any given machine to any other, and to relate all machines to the prime purposes of diagnosis and therapy.

The very words "diagnosis" and "therapy" symbolize the

nominal and unreal divisions that history has forced upon us and that continue to trap us to this day. In the 18th century, doctors had thousands of remedies for diseases they could not accurately recognize. The 19th century went into praiseworthy reaction—which, as in so many other fields, it overdid: no remedy should be attempted, was the rule, until an accurate diagnosis had been made. The pendulum swung too far, and diagnosis became an end in itself. The great men of medicine had but one function: to pin down disease with the same superior mastery that Sherlock Holmes displayed in pinning down criminals. Once the great men had spoken, the management of the patient could be left to lesser men, as Holmes left his criminals to the slower-witted police. In many fields this unhealthy division between diagnosis and therapy (even between treatment and after-care) persists today.

What is diagnosis? It is a process for extracting information from a complex, interdependent, intercommunicating set of physical and chemical events (i.e. life—the reason for resorting to this cumbersome definition will soon become clear). And therapy? It is a process for changing those same events so that they either revert to a normal pattern or assume a new state of equilibrium. In short, these two elements correspond to the two processes we can discern in *any* complex control circuit: feedback and control. Both are fundamentally involved in the handling of information—inward and outward bound. (It is hard to think of a spoonful of medicine as "information," but that, in our present context, is exactly what it is.) To ensure that we are not now pursuing a mere analogy, we need only look at the power levels involved in each element.

In any cybernetic system it is of the essence that the energy consumed by the sensing elements (thermostats, voltmeters, rev counters, etc.) should be minute compared with the energy consumed to maintain or change the system. Thermostats do actually cool the rooms that house them, but I should not envy the man who set out to measure the loss to the room. Similarly in diagnosis we find that those methods that rely on physiological energy consume a minute proportion of it. An EKG diagnosis, for instance, consumes energy in the microjoule range to measure a single heartbeat. (I refer, of course, to the electrical energy that, tapped from the body and amplified, moves the EKG writer. Left to itself this energy is dissipated in random thermal movements that fractionally raise the body's temperature.) The heartbeat itself consumes between 40 and 400 joules, and the therapeutic restarting of the heart consumes 300 joules of energy in one powerful shock. These relationships between the energy demands of the feedback and command circuits are characteristic of all efficient self-regulating systems.

In short, the entity that unites both diagnosis and therapy is *information*; and, it turns out, this same entity provides that fundamental unifying concept I mentioned earlier. Life is a system *obsessed* with information. The genes that control our growth, our defenses, our susceptibilities—and often, too, our manner of death—are no more than four chemicals of a particular architecture arranged in particular sequences that constitute a code. They operate, in turn, through molecules (enzymes) of a precise architecture that determines both mode and speed of interaction. Thus the network of chemical pathways we call *metabolism* is the information network of a homeostat. *Even in sickness it remains an efficient network*; to be sure, it is then processing wrong information or using wrong channels, but it is nonetheless a functioning network. Only in terminal states, when the volume of informational traffic falls below the critical volume that makes for a self-sustaining, living organism, do the strands of the network begin to fall apart.

Medical machines are adjuncts to this information network. They work either by extending existing channels (as in biochemical analysis) or by providing new channels, unknown in nature (as in all electrograph machines). By classifying these channels—or, more strictly, the arenas within which these channels are linked—we arrive at a kind of spectrum, somewhere along which any given machine can be placed.

Such a spectrum is shown on page 162. Obviously many more subdivisions could be made, but, because the idea of classifying medical machines in this way will be novel to many, I have kept it down to four simple arenas. The first two relate to the familiar macroscopic world, the world we can manipulate in real time and

	A	B	C	D
ARENA	Macrosystems in direct contact	Macrosystems acting at a distance	Microsystems	Molecular systems
CHANNEL	Pressure & manipulation	Sound & electricity	Vision	Chemical activity
FEEDBACK IN THERAPY	ABCD	AB	None	ABCD
USUAL MODE	On-line and real time	On-line and real time	Off-line	Off-line
SUBJECT	Large systems	Large and microscopic systems	Microscopic cell communities	Molecular activity of cell communities
EXAMPLES *(non-machine activities in italics)*	*Feeling* Sphygmomanometer Thermometer Spirometer Manometer Ballistocardiogram All surgery Dental surgery Massage Physiotherapy All prostheses Heart-lung machine Artificial kidney Respirator Iron lung Contraceptive devices	*Patient's own words* *visual inspection* *percussion* Stethoscope EKG EEG EMG Audiometer Electromagnetic blood flow meter Ultrasound devices Myoelectric stimulus ECT Defibrillation Pacemakers EEG anesthesia Psychotherapy Radio pills Labeled isotopes Short-wave diathermy Radiant heat Laser applications UV devices X ray therapy Gamma ray therapy	histology biopsy immunization	biochemistry hematology chemotherapy

watch the resultant activity. The second two cover the microscopic and quantum arenas, where the real biological action is but where our approach is clumsy and circuitous. The contrast between the two could hardly be greater. We have a vast range of machines that operate in real time at the macroscopic level—a level at which it is really quite impossible to manipulate the bionetwork in any but the grossest ways; and we have slow, cumbersome, off-line machines (none therapeutic) that let us probe the mysteries of that network, but not in real time.

The nature of biological activity places fundamental limits on the improvements we can make at the macrosystem level. It is my guess that we are close to a state of diminishing returns already. That is to say, we can make machines handier, more stable, more reliable, but, great though these advances may be, they will not yield fundamentally new kinds of information about the human organism. For instance, we shall probably soon be able to make EKG's that will slip into a vest pocket and yet be sophisticated enough to monitor the heartbeat of an at-risk patient and give him 2 or 3 hours' warning of an impending attack (or, at least, of those attacks that signal their onset in EKG abnormalities prior to the actual attack). Such an advance would be an enormous benefit to tens of thousands of heart sufferers, and I would not for a moment suggest that we should not pursue it and similar developments with all our vigor. Nothing in this chapter should be construed as an attempt to throw cold water on improvements in instrumentation. But we delude ourselves if we think that ultimate progress lies along a path strewn with piecemeal advances in physics and engineering. Our real hopes, surely, must be pinned on chemistry, which until recently was the Cinderella of bio-engineering.

All the activities we call "living" are under chemical (i.e. genetic) control. In a recent remarkable book (see Suggested Reading), Dr. Philip Burch has shown that many conditions not previously thought to have a significant genetic component—

Opposite: machines and activities from many aspects of medical practice are displayed in relation to the arenas in which they operate. Such a classification shows very clearly our inability to probe the biological information network at the cellular and molecular levels.

such as dental caries, coronary thrombosis, diabetes, and bone fractures—have a genetic basis. Indeed, it is probable that growth, disease, and aging are all aspects of the same genetic process. If so, the prospects for medical progress are bright indeed. For we no longer think of the genes as being locked away in some unattainable mendelian fastness; we know plenty of chemicals that can get at them—all, alas, harmful—but nevertheless it shows that the genes are not beyond our reach. We know, too, that natural pathways exist for turning the genes on and off, as it were. The most stupendous example of this is in the pair of pictures on page 152. The frog in the upper picture was produced by the mating-spawning-metamorphosing process that has evolved over millions of years. But every cell in the frog in the lower picture is the progeny of a freak. The man who helped "create" this frog, Dr. J. B. Gurdon of Oxford University, removed the nucleus from the original egg and replaced it with the nucleus of a cell taken from the intestine of an already advanced tadpole— that is, from a cell already highly specialized. The characteristics of the resulting frog are thus determined entirely by a nucleus taken from a specialized cell. The fact that the frog is in every way indistinguishable from others of its species shows that all the information needed for the development of an entire organism is contained in the nucleus of every cell in that organism's body. And from this it follows that during specialization, cells do not lose genetic information, but merely switch off the genes they do not need (in practice, most of the genes are thus switched off). Dr. Gurdon's experiment shows that, in at least one set of circumstances (nuclear transplantation), *all* those genes can be reactivated. From other studies we know that genes can be diverted from their purpose (this is how viruses persuade our cells to stop making normal protein and to replicate viruses instead) and that they can change during life (the genetic abnormalities of cancer being an example).

To sum up: all biological activity is under genetic control, and genes can be diverted, modified, and switched on and off. Here is the basis for fundamental advance in bio-engineering. Only from such premises can we develop the machines that will fill out the two threadbare columns of our spectrum—and enable

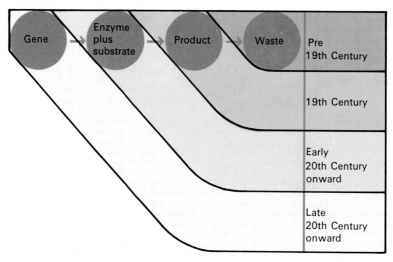

The diagram above relates the main stages of biochemical activity to our growing skill at monitoring them (see text).

us to delete "off-line" and substitute "on-line and real time."

Meanwhile...

The knowledge that our ultimate goal is to be achieved through chemical rather than physical means should help us direct our efforts and apply our resources along the most fruitful lines. Obviously we cannot yet specify (or even imagine) the machines that will accomplish changes at the microscopic and molecular level in real time. We have a great deal to do before we can think of such a specification. To start with, we need to know vastly more about normal physiology at the most detailed biochemical level. Historically our investigations have followed the scheme outlined in the diagram above. This relates the four major stages of biochemical production to our growing skill at measuring that activity. Basically those four stages show a decreasing complexity (for good thermodynamic reasons, because the entropy increases at each stage). As you would expect, we have approached this problem beginning at the easy end: the waste products.

With growing skill and confidence we have advanced to the walls of the inner citadel itself: the genetic control center. At each stage of gathering complexity the rewards to be reaped have increased many-fold. The subtlety of our approach has also increased.

Already we are learning to see ill health not as a single, special category but as a collective name for a number of variants of the bioprocess itself; and like many collective names it is useful at only the grossest level. A similar change took place in mental health at the turn of the century, when clinically unhelpful categories such as *mad, evil, possessed* were exchanged for more informative terms. Hence comes our need to know more about this state we call *normal*.

In Chapter 3, I also mentioned this need to define normality more tightly than at present, but I spoke merely in terms of individual patients and normal ranges. In this present, more broadly based, chapter, I must add that merely to know the normal ranges in individuals—invaluable though it would be— is not nearly enough. We must also correlate these ranges with one another. In a decade or so, it will be considered inferior practice to diagnose or treat a patient (except in emergency) without a full biochemical profile at least. In time such profiles will come to include personality, aptitudes, preferences, habits, disease patterns—any factor that shows some significant relationship. And in case you may doubt the value of such profiles let me say that if we could achieve them today, even though we made no matching advance in diagnosis or therapy, we could at least double the efficiency of medicine by any yardstick you might care to choose.

As an example, lung cancer correlates with smoking. Everybody knows that. How many people know that lung cancer also correlates significantly with coffee drinking, with sugar intake, with the eating of spicy food, with sexual intercourse, with body type, with personality, with emotional type? There must be many other factors that we cannot measure—especially the genes, which are at the heart of this correlation. The genes are the predisposing factors, and some of the other correlations are multipliers—including smoking, far and away the most powerful multiplier of all. As doctors, in our present state of ignorance, we are justified in a blanket of condemnation of smoking; we are right to advise every patient to give it up. But as biologists we must be fascinated by the fact that some are much more susceptible than others—with the possibility that there may be some patients who could smoke 60 a day all their lives and yet live a full life without developing lung cancer, bronchitis, emphysema, heart disease, or any of the other ailments that correlate with smoking. In the same way there may be patients who can gorge on cholesterol-rich foods, grow fat as lard, and never suffer a hint of arterial or coronary trouble—just as there are patients who do all the right things and yet fall victim to everything that's going.

The ancient response to this seeming injustice—a shrug of the shoulders, a few muttered words about there being more things in heaven and earth, etc.—is beginning to wear thin. We grow daily more aware that the onset of disease or disorder is not a stochastic event; no cosmic dice rattle out our fates in the simple way we could once believe. Almost all disease, we now see, is multifactorial in much the same way as the smoking/lung cancer correlation is multifactorial. If we could pin down those factors for each disease we could begin to turn medicine into a truly predictive science. We could say to a patient, for instance: "Your chances of getting such and such a disease are so remote that you can forget them. However, people of your profile stand a 40-per-cent chance of getting such and such; you can more than halve that chance by doing the following things . . ." and so on. You can imagine the colossal statistical analyses that will be needed to back up such a medicine, but you will also appreciate the gain in efficiency—we could, for instance, single out at-risk patients much earlier and much more certainly than at present.

But we shall not understand the mechanism of disease until we apply this new insight in every field of medicine—especially in our habitual ways of talking (and thus of thinking) about it. We still say, for instance, that colds are *caused* by viruses; in fact, colds merely correlate highly with virus invasion, but not vice versa—that is, not all virus invasions lead to colds, even among people who have no antibodies against the viruses in question. Why do such people not catch cold, despite their lack of orthodox defense? If we *really* understood disease, we should have no difficulty in framing an answer. The fact that we cannot answer is just another aspect of the lamentably backward state of modern medicine.

Yet we can at least pinpoint the deficiencies with fair accuracy; and we can map the path along which improvements must lie—in fact, I have done so for the first few stages. When we know what correlates, positively or negatively, and what does not correlate, we can begin to ask "why" questions with some certainty that the answers exist. Already, for instance, we can ask why extraverts with strong libidos, excitable tempers, and a taste for rich foods and cigarettes are far more likely to get lung cancer than are unemotional, undersexed introverts who like plain food and do not smoke? We can ask this question because an enormous amount of research has been done on this one disease. When similar studies of other diseases and conditions have been made (and many are now in progress) we can even begin to correlate the questions! We shall see patterns that we cannot now suspect. And the patterns will suggest mechanisms, the mechanisms will generate theories, the theories will demand testing—and this will call for new generations of machines. And in this way, too, the empty columns in our spectrum of machines will slowly be filled.

Power = Responsibility

Perhaps before the turn of this century we shall be able to crack and re-form the molecules on which life depends with the same ease that we now have in cracking and re-forming far simpler organic compounds in oil refineries. How shall we use such power? In less change-ridden days we could safely leave such questions to be sorted out in the fullness of time. Revolutions happened only once a generation, if that. Men had time to accommodate to change. Today's senior doctors have survived three revolutions (chemotherapy, electronics, and plastics) with considerably less ease. How many will today's medical students have to endure in our half-thinking fashion? Of one thing we can be certain: the pace is already too fast for problems to "sort themselves out in their own way." Machines have already posed us some dreadful choices—choices that our ethical traditions cannot clearly answer.

For example, there was a time when if you had a flat EEG, no heart beat, and no spontaneous sign of breathing, you would have been dead by any reckoning. Today you can show all three signs and yet live. Your heart can be restarted (many times if necessary) with a defibrillator; your breathing can be provided or assisted by a mechanical respirator; and your EEG may spontaneously return even after a fortnight of EEG silence. People have recovered from such a state to lead perfectly normal lives. The dilemma is posed not by them but by those who are not taken to the defibrillator and the respirator in time to save their brains from irreparable damage. The machines save their bodies but not their brains. The resulting "vegetables," as they are sometimes called, have to be fed (they will eat only by reflex as the food touches their tongue), washed, turned, and tended in every function. They can live (if that is the word) like this for 20 years or more. But for the machines, they would certainly be dead. Are they, then, alive?

This is not a question to be answered by looking up "life" in a dictionary. The definition of, and statements about, life that I have used in this book are, even for me, no guide here, for they were not intended to apply in this context. The convenient pigeon-holes of biology, or of law, were not intended for the messy world of distressed relatives, of hospitals short of staff and beds. In *that* world, like it or not, we first decide whether we want to call such vegetables living, and frame our definitions accordingly.

But if two simple machines such as a respirator and a defibrillator can cause such a problem, what are we to expect from the promethean machines of the years to come? Those machines will not leave us hanging uncertainly between life and death; they will confer powers that, to us, seem godlike. It is fruitless to try to guess how they will seem to doctors and patients who are probably not yet born.

In ethics each of us is the child of his age. There is no profit in resolving dilemmas that do not yet exist. If the people of the future want to use these powerful machines for purposes that most of us would regard as wrong, dangerous, or perverted, it will be their problem, not ours. Certainly, like all advances of great potential benefit, the machines will have great capacity for evil, too. I can only end by saying how I should hope to use them if I lived that long. And, like everyone who delivers an ethical opinion, I like to feel that my morality springs from something more than the local needs and customs of my own time. It is possibly a delusion, but I should like to foster it by going back three centuries for one of its most perfect expressions, in Dryden's *Oedipus*, the play he wrote with Nathaniel Lee:

"Of no distemper, of no blast he died,
But fell like autumn-fruit that mellowed long,
Ev'n wondered at because he dropp'd no sooner.
Fate seemed to wind him up for fourscore years
Yet freely ran he on ten winters more;
'Till, like a clock worn out with eating time,
The weary wheels of life at last stood still."

Any medical worker would surely be proud to have helped offer such a life and such a way of going to anyone who wanted it.

Machines in Use

In writing this book I have frequently had to stifle the impulse to mention as many machines as possible. I know many readers will have bought this book expecting a sort of mini-encyclopedia of medical machinery. To satisfy both (that is, the impulse I bottled so frequently as well as the readers my title may have misled) I have appended this glossary of 125 machines.

Even so, despite the condensation that a glossary style makes possible, I have still been forced to select rather drastically. I have had to exclude, for instance, all hospital catering equipment, furniture, architectural fittings, information systems, and surgical instruments. The remaining machines fall into two broad categories already discussed in the main body of the book: diagnostic and therapeutic. There is a third category, research machinery, which is by nature a temporary label. At one time every machine listed here was a research machine.

The resulting list has two major defects, temporal and personal. It is out of date as soon as it is written, such is the breakneck progress of biomedical engineering; the defect is inherent in the subject itself, so I need make no apology. It is also *my* list. It suffers from my limited knowledge and it reveals my blind spots. For this I must apologize. Nevertheless I hope enough has filtered through to have made the effort worth the while.

▲ = diagnostic, ● = research, ■ = therapeutic. Of course all diagnostic and to a lesser extent therapeutic machines are used as research tools.

■ Air sterilization

The ideal operating theater and the postoperative transplant area need completely sterile air around the patient. This can be achieved by filtration down to 0.3 microns and injecting the resulting pure air in a curtain around the patient.

■ Anal plug, electronic

Device for promoting anal continence. Held by anal sphincter and pelvic floor, it delivers a tetanizing (contracting) stimulus through electrodes on its surface. Stimulator (pinned on clothes) give 1 ms. impulse at the rate of 200/min—up to 12 v. Battery lasts 7 days.

▲ Angiograph

Used to investigate arteries and veins. Radio-opaque liquid injected upstream is filmed on a series of X-ray exposures. Flow patterns can also be established by injecting radio-isotopes and counting downstream. Lymph angiograms can be done by locating lymphatics with an injection of dye, which is taken up by the lymph vessels, following this with a slow injection of radio-opaque medium.

● Artificial heart

Rubber and plastic and metal pumps to support circulation whilst waiting for transplant. Power sources, clotting, reliability, incorporation, and output remain as problems. (Lengthy discussion in *Spare-Part Surgery*.)

■ Artificial kidney

An extracorporeal circulation machine connected as an arterio-venous or veno-venous circuit. Either relies on arterio-venous pressure drop to move blood or incorporates a pump. Consists essentially of a membrane with small pores, blood at pressure on one side, and dialyzing fluid on the other. Wastes in blood diffuse through pores into fluid. Membrane can be in flat sheets or coiled tubes.

▲ Audiometer

Measurable noise emitter to assess auditory perception. Volume and frequency can be varied independently to determine precise degree of hearing ability.

■ Autoclave

Term used for enclosed sterilizing container. May use dry heat, steam, or humidified ethylene oxide combined with pressure as the sterilizing agents. Various cycles of operation—sometimes with a partial vacuum to dry off excess moisture or to remove ethylene oxide. Heat remains the best agent for materials that will stand it.

▲ Automatic analyzers

Machines that automate biochemical analysis and give readouts that can be either interpreted by an operator or fed onto computer cards. Examples are AutoAnalyzer, Multichannel 300, Autolab, Analmatic, Bioanalyst, Clinomac, Mecolab, and Autochemist.

▲● Ballistocardiograph

A machine to measure the "recoil" of the ejecting heart. May use damped suspension to support the patient on a platform or use air-cushion frictionless suspension. Gives useful indication of degree of coordination in heart contraction. Unique among cardiological measurements in that it has *predictive* value—e.g. of the likelihood of coronary attack.

▲ Bed weigher

In some diseases and metabolic studies and in renal dialysis it is often necessary to weigh a bedbound and perhaps unconscious patient frequently and accurately. The best weighers use hydraulic bed legs and measure the hydraulic fluid pressure.

▲ Bicycle Ergometer

A simple device using a bicycle-like machine in which pedal load can be exactly specified. Patients do measured exercises during EKG, respiratory, or cardiovascular studies.

▲ Bladder controller, electrical

Device to promote urinary continence. Platinum electrodes from implanted radio receiver carry tetanizing (contracting) stimulus to bladder-sphincter muscle. Battery-powered transmitter, carried externally, is switched off to relax sphincter and allow micturition. Can be used as a pessary to avoid surgery.

■● Blind navigational aids

Various methods exist enabling blind people to recognize light from dark, proximity of objects, color, etc. Some use reflective light onto photocell with audible warning, others use the echo principle. An experimental device uses a matrix of microvibrators connected to a small TV camera; light and dark areas are converted to vibrating and still areas, which can be sensed by nerves in skin.

▲● Blood flow probe

Usually involves putting a magnet and coil around a blood vessel; blood (an ionized fluid in motion) generates currents in the coil; requires surgery through a magnetic field. On the same principle there is an implantable intravascular flow meter in a 2.2-mm. catheter 1 m. long. In peripheral muscle, which is constantly cooling and is constantly reheated by incoming blood, one can measure local changes of flow by noting minute local temperature

changes. System uses semiconductor devices in circuits compensated to eliminate effects of whole-body temperature rise.

■ Blood loss monitor

Device to assess blood lost in swabs etc. during surgery. Articles containing blood are put into an agitated container and measurement is by electrical conductivity or by colorimeter.

▲ Blood oxygen cell

An oxygen electrode whose electrical output measures the oxygen tension of the solution in which it is placed.

● Blood pressure monitor

The patient-borne monitor is a direct-writing, clock-driven instrument worn under the coat. Sensor, worn on thumb under a thumb stall, is an inflatable cuff coupled to a servo-mechanism that maintains suitable cuff pressure. Regularly timed dots on a chart record systolic pressure for up to 24 hours.

▲ Blood pressure transducers

1. Large types ($\frac{3}{4}''$ to $1''$ dia., $1\frac{1}{2}''$ long) use strain gauge, or variably occluded grid with photocell, or variable resistance (=microphone).
2. Small types (down to less than 1 mm.) are semiconductor strain gauges.

▲ Blood volume computer

One method of assessing the patient's blood volume is to inject a substance that remains in the blood compartment and does not diffuse throughout the body. It is then possible to take a sample of blood after sufficient time has elapsed for full mixing and to assess the dilution of the sample. The most accurate method is to use a radioisotope. Three counts are made: (1) On the patient's basal blood radiation and background irradiation; (2) From a known volume of the isotope that is to be injected; and (3) On a blood sample from the patient after mixing has taken place. A blood volume computer then gives the blood volume with high accuracy assuming it has not changed and that the isotope has remained in the blood compartment. Usually these assumptions are invalid.

■ Blood warming coil

Stored blood for transfusion is usually kept at 4°c. Patients who receive large transfusions may be considerably cooled and the heart fibrillates. Special coils are available immersed in water baths to heat blood before transfusion. Coils for immersion in heart-lung machines are also available to act as heat exchangers.

▲ Breath test meter

Gets maximum information from one forced expiration. Computes FEV1, vital capacity, and peak flow (all described in the text) from pressure changes on a porous diaphragm of gauze. *See also* Respiration monitor.

▲● Calorimeter

A device for measuring the quantity of heat absorbed or emitted from a substance during a known temperature change. From this can be calculated its thermal capacity. Used in metabolic studies on food—e.g. calorific values.

● Cancer cell centrifuge

Centrifuge that separates heavy cell nuclei (which may be cancerous) from more normal light ones. Cells are collected from cervical smears, peritoneal fluid, etc.

▲ Cardiac monitor

Many forms of cardiac monitor are used, ranging from simple EKG radio meters to complex monitors that sound alarms with rhythm changes and incorporate memory loops so that a study of what had preceded the rhythm change may be made.

■ Cardiac press

A lever system for making easier external cardiac massage—which can be hard physical work. Some are manual, some oxygen-or-air-powered, with an automatic attachment for ventilating the patient.

▲●■ Cathode-ray tube

Commonly used for displaying electrocardiograms, electroencephalograms and the monitoring of most physiological parameters. It is also used in conjunction with computer terminals. Its great advantage is that the electron beam has negligible inertia—a factor that can distort readings from recorders with moving arms or mirrors.

■● Cell filters

Filters with minute pores of precisely determined size. They can be used, for example, to separate cancer cells from blood. Some can be placed within the syringe that withdraws the blood.

▲ Centrifuge

Clinical centrifuges take 100 ml. samples up to 25,000 rpm in 45 sec. with temperature ranges between -20 and $+40$°c. They are used to separate light and heavy components of physiological fluids—e.g. cells from blood.

▲● Clinical steroid analyzer

High speed gas chromatograph set up for urinary 17-ketosteroids to diagnose gland disturbances involving ketosteroid metabolism.

▲ Clot timer

A small capillary tube containing a metal ball. This tube can be mechanically rocked backward and forward and the time taken for stopping the ball, recorded automatically, gives an index of the clotting time.

▲ Colony counter

The counting of bacterial colonies on

a plate can be difficult and tedious because of their lack of symmetry. A colony counter has a special illumination system and a means of marking colonies that have been counted, so that the operator can mark off the colonies one at a time; the counting is automatically recorded.

▲ **Colorimeter**
A device for comparing the color of a substance (usually a solution) with a standard reference. Used usually for chemical analysis.

▲● **Color TV endoscopy**
Used for peritoneal examination, usually in gynecology. Consists of a 16-inch-long probe the diameter of a pencil with a fiber optic light guide and a lens attached to a TV camera and an ordinary color TV monitor. Enables the surgeon to examine and discuss the condition of abdominal viscera.

▲ **Computing spirometer**
A simple device for measuring the amount of air breathed in and out under various respiratory situations. Computing spirometers have electromechanical devices to do the calculations for the doctor. (*See also* Breath test meter, Pulmonary function analyzer, Respiration monitor.)

▲ **Continuous integrator**
Electric integration of signals from different measuring instruments allowing, for example, the peaks of a densitometer and chromatograph to be integrated giving usable information instantly; without such an aid the information might not be available in time.

▲ **Cryostat**
Thermostatically maintained cold bed for frozen sections and blades of microtomes.

■● **Cryosurgical tools**
Devices for freezing and killing small or large areas of tissue while severing fewer vessels than in traditional surgery. Dead areas are removed by natural process. Also used to harden very soft tissue before certain kinds of conventional surgery. Chiefly used in skin, eye, brain, and tumor surgery.

■ **Cryotherm limb cooler**
Refrigerator unit connected to special "blankets" to cool limbs and reduce metabolism before and during surgery.

■ **Deaf aids**
Battery - driven microphone - and - amplifier systems that conduct augmented sound either through the natural ear channels or through the bone of the skull. Special mains-driven devices with tone selection are used in education.

■ **Decompression units**
Used on divers with "the bends" and for the treatment of air embolism following heart-lung surgery. If the patient is compressed in a high-pressure atmosphere of pure oxygen, intravascular bubbles (which, in fact, consist of nitrogen), are re-dissolved; subsequent slow decompression allows these excess gases to diffuse out naturally without bubbling and so relieves the patient. (*See also* Hyperbaric chamber.)

■ **Defibrillator**
Device for restarting a fibrillating (writhing) heart. In open chest surgery, where the electrodes can be placed directly on the heart, a direct-current discharge is normally used with 20 joules for children and 30-50 for adults. The discharge wire has a special form with a slow build-up to prevent the rapid energy changes that damage the heart muscle. (Alternating current defibrillators are now obsolete.) With external defibrillation (chest closed) a

6000-8000 volt shock is used with total energies up to 400 joules. Double defibrillation, using a carefully timed second shock 85-100 milliseconds after the first to depolarize those muscle fibers that were not depolarized by the first discharge, is aimed at reducing total energy requirements and makes it possible to externally defibrillate with total energies of only 20-40 joules. Loss of heart efficiency (which usually follows high-power defibrillation) is minimized.

■ **Dental pulp tester**
An electric nerve-stimulating device for testing the thickness of dentine lying over the pulp of a tooth; if it is thin, even a weak stimulus is felt.

▲● **Dewar flask**
A double-walled glass vessel. The space between the walls is evacuated and the walls themselves usually coated with a metallic highly reflecting surface. The purpose of the flask is to emulate its contents thermally, to keep them hot or cold at a steady temperature.

■ **Dialyzate supply unit**
Various forms of dialyzate supply units exist, mostly consisting of proportioning pumps. Some are connected to peritoneal dialysis units, which pass measured amounts of dialyzing fluid into the peritoneal cavity, suck it out to waste, and repeat the process, in order to give automatic peritoneal dialysis.

▲● **Doppler rheograph**
Ultrasound emitter and receiver for measuring movement and velocity by comparing frequencies of emitted and reflected waves (Doppler shift). Can be used to detect fetal pulse at 10-12 weeks by reflection from moving fetus. Also reveals blood velocity in superficial vessels.

■ **Dosimeter**
Disks of radiation-sensitive thermo-luminescent phosphors combined in teflon plastic. When removed and heated they emit light whose intensity corresponds to cumulative radiation exposure discharge signals. (*See also* Radiation monitor.)

▲● **Echo pill**
Radio pill using tuned not battery powered circuit. (*See also* Radio pill.)

● **Electrical skin tester**
Device to test for possible lung cancer by measuring chest's electrical resistance. Such resistance depends in part on conduction along sympathetic nerves, and it rises slowly if these nerves are compressed or damaged (by, for example, a lung cancer).

▲● **Electrocardiogram waveform monitor**
Device that detects rhythm changes in an EKG, which may predict or even indicate a heart attack; can be set to give audible or visual warning.

▲ **Electrocardiograph (EKG)**
Device for recording electrical activity of heart muscle. Electrodes lead from limbs and points on chest; comparison of varying potentials between specific electrodes reveals electrical state of heart. Writers use ink, heat, or ultra-violet light on special papers. To avoid psychological interference with the record the Mediscreen chair has contact EKG electrodes in the arms and seat and records EKG (and pulse and respiratory rate) unbeknown to its user.

▲ **Electroencephalograph (EEG)**
Sensitive multichannel meter and writing device to detect electrical activity of the brain. Each area has its own characteristic rhythms, disturbances of which may be diagnostically significant.

▲ **Electrophoresis**

A method of sorting out various substances in plasma utilizing their property of different speeds of migration in an electric field; usually done along strips of blotting paper; may be done on a surface of a gel. One refinement, electrofocusing, is used for analytical separation of proteins according to their isoelectric points. Complete separation can be made if difference is as small as 0.0002 pH units. Low-molecular-weight carrier amphocytes (proteins) are exposed to a voltage in a convection-free medium. A natural pH gradient forms. Large-molecular-weight amphocytes (also proteins) will concentrate in narrow bands corresponding to their specific isoelectric point, pI.

▲ **Electromyograph (EMG)**

Device similar to EKG for recording electrical potential associated with muscular activity. Used in study of nervous and muscular disorders.

▲● **Electronic sphygmomanometer**

Conventional blood-pressure armband with built-in crystal microphone, signals from which operate lights whose appearance and disappearance show systolic and diastolic pressures.

▲ **Electronic stethoscope**

Used either by deaf doctors who require amplification or as a teaching instrument so that a large number of people may listen to one heart.

▲● **Electrosleep unit**

Electronarcosis is a development of electrocortical therapy (once common). Properly controlled electrical stimulation of the brain causes unconsciousness that passes into sleep. EEG readings suggest that relaxation is usually poor. Safety is uncertain.

▲● **Ellipsometer**

Device for measuring the optical thickness of films from a few angstroms up to a few thousand angstroms thick. It provides a new and quick method to determine the strength of an immunological reaction. Antigen-coated slides are placed in a solution of the patient's blood serum (which can be diluted a millionfold) and antigen-antibody reaction is promoted by electric current. The amount of antibody adsorbed onto the slide indicates the strength of the reaction. Even if it is only a few angstroms thick it can still be measured accurately.

■● **Endarterectomy**

Technique for stripping out of atheroma (a fatty substance) that blocks or partially blocks an artery.

Drills: Various drill ends attached to catheters have been tried as a method of reboring arteries. They vary in pattern from simple corkscrews to complex devices resembling oil well drills.

Gas: A needle-fine jet of high-pressure CO_2 has been used to strip the atheroma from vessel walls.

Laser: Laser light carried through fiber-optic light guides can selectively destroy atheroma.

▲ **Endocamera**

Attached to various forms of endoscope in order to keep a permanent record, particularly useful in bronchoscopy.

▲ **Endoscope**

To look into the stomach and other body cavities, it is sometimes necessary to have a flexible instrument. The simplest devices for achieving this are fiber-optic light guides (although internal gold-plated tubes acting as light guides can be as effective).

■● **Enuresis control unit**

Device to control bed-wetting. It relies on the fact that wetting the bed can be cured by waking the subject up every time it happens in order that a reflex can be established for them to wake at the appropriate times. One way to do this is to use a low voltage grid of wires so arranged that when urine passes on to them it makes an electrical contact which sounds an alarm to wake the patient.

A further attachment can stop flow of urine after first drop (which triggers the device) either by inflating a balloon against the pelvic floor or by electrical stimulus of muscles in the pelvic floor.

▲ **Eye testing unit**

Uses opthalmometer, coincidence refractionometer and slit lamp and smaller instruments in a rotating support clamped to patient's head.

▲●■ **Fiber optics (light guide)**

If two concentric cylinders of glass of different refractive indices are heated so that they are nearly melted, they can be drawn out into an extremely fine glass fiber with a completely internal reflecting sheath.Thousands of such fibers, gathered coherently form a flexible light guide that gives good optical definition.

■ **Fibrillator**

Device for causing the heart to fibrillate—for example, during surgery to avoid the entrance of air into the blood system. A small AC current with a potential of up to 12 volts is sufficient. Normal beating usually resumes when switched off. Otherwise conventional defibrillation is used.

▲ **Fluorimeter**

Many chemical solutions when irradiated with visible or ultraviolet light absorb the light and re-emit light of a different wavelength. Fluorescence of

this type can be used for analysis, of, for example, vitamins and steroids. Can use mercury and zinc lamps.

■● **Freeze dryer (lyophilizer)**

Device for drying frozen tissues by sublimation of ice to vapor in a vacuum. "Flash" (rapid) freezing prevents ice crystal formation and damage due to excessive concentration of solutes at end of freezing. Used in histology and skin banks. (*See* Cryostat.)

▲● **Heartrate telemeter**

Most cardiac arrests in people with damaged heart muscle can be prevented by treating rhythm disturbances before arrest occurs. To detect those disturbances the patient wears an electrocardiograph, the rhythm of which is transmitted by a small portable radio transmitter to a central radio receiving center, where changes are analyzed.

■ **Humidifier**

Patients who breathe through tubes need humid air, since the natural humidifier (nose and pharynx) is bypassed. Humidifiers use atomizers ("perfume sprays"), evaporators, or ultrasound atomization. Humid air (42% relative humidity) is also needed in ethylene oxide sterilization.

■ **Hyperbaric chamber**

High-pressure chamber used for increasing oxygen content of a given volume of blood. Operating type is large enough to contain surgeons and patient. Portable bed type is used for coronary care, gas gangrene, and embolism. Pressure is usually 3 atmospheres absolute. Fire risk precludes all electrical devices except rigorously tested intercom. High pressure makes tumors more sensitive to irradiation and is used as an adjunct to radiotherapy. Also used in routine decompression among divers. Leaks and sudden decompression can damage the ears.

■● Hyper/hypothermia machine

Refrigerator for whole body cooling to 30°c by means of wrap-around water blankets. Its use protects bone marrow from damage when cytotoxic drugs are used in cancer therapy. Rewarming, by passing warm water through blankets, is slower because possible temperature gradient is smaller; tissues burn above 43°c.

■ Hypodermic filter

Millipore filter for use with hypodermic injectors to sterilize fluids from multi-dose vials, radio-isotopes, etc. which carry a risk of infection; 0.45 or 0.22 micron pore size; 25 or 13 mm. diameter to fit syringe.

▲ Image intensifier

Electronic tube multiplies strength of available light up to 1,000,000 times. Made of sandwich of phosphor/photo-cathodes with 20 line pairs/mm. using magnetic focusing trialkali S.20 photo-cathodes. Makes it possible to reduce X-ray dosage without loss of image.

● Impedance cardiogram

Changes of electrical impedance across the chest provide a continuous qualitative record of changes in heart size. Uses standard EKG skin electrodes. Display is on any vector cardioscope in two planes or XY plotter.

▲ Infrared gas analyzer

Measures CO_2 in human breath cycle from color changes in infrared absorption spectrum (CO_2 is a powerful absorber of infrared).

■● Labor decompression unit

A deflatable plastic tent placed around a pregnant mother's abdomen for brief spells during pregnancy and before labor to reduce blood pressure around abdomen (and hence fetus) to 70 mm. Hg. Aids blood flow to uterus and baby; leads to easier labor—and possibly brighter babies.

▲● Labor monitor

Unit for monitoring fetal and maternal conditions during labor. It records: intra-uterine pressure, fetal EKG, fetal heart rate, and electro-myogram of uterus. Can be set to sound alarm when preset rates are exceeded or unmet.

■● Larynx, electronic

Pulse generator held against throat to make "noise" which can be modified by nose, mouth, etc. With training it can make a near-normal voice in a laryngectomized patient.

■● Laser

Various forms of laser have been used medically. The commonest one is the ruby laser stimulated by very powerful neon flash tubes. Q-switched lasers in which the pulse is "compressed" in time have been used in detached retina operations but have proved harmful; the extremely rapid dissipation of energy produces a shock wave that mechanically damages the inside of the eye. Gas lasers, CO_2 etc. may also be used. (*See also* Endarterectomy.)

▲ Mass spectrometer

A device for identifying the elements of a substance by producing a high velocity stream of ions from the substance and deflecting them by a magnetic field. The amount by which the various particles are deflected depends upon their mass and the resulting distribution of the ions permits their identification.

▲● Medical telemetry

Various radiotelemetry devices, implantable, swallowable, and wearable are available; the 102.2—102.4 MHz band is reserved for this purpose. Two recently announced transmit blood pressure and EKG rhythms, a boon to patients at risk from rhythm disturbances. (*See also* Radio pill.)

● **Microcapsules**

Microcapsules have ultrathin membranes (200 angstrom, permeable only to smaller molecules). 10 ml. of 20-micron microcapsules have a total surface area of 2500 cm², rather more than that of a conventional artificial kidney. Theoretical studies show that microcapsules loaded with the right enzymes and mixed with suitable ion-exchange resins could duplicate many kidney functions.

● **Microdensitometer**

Device for measuring optical density at different points of microscope specimens. Used for determining presence and size of cell constituents. The light absorbed by a stain in a sample is proportional to the mass of the cell and can give an accurate measure of, for instance, relative amounts of DNA.

▲ **Micromanipulator**

Device for manipulation under microscope with position accuracy of 10 microns.

▲● **Microscopes**

In theory objects less than ½ a wavelength apart cannot be separated. In practice, magnification greater than 2000× is difficult to achieve with optical systems. The ordinary light microscope is a basic tool used in practically every laboratory for counting blood cells, for examining routine histological specimens and for many other purposes. The limitations of an optical system lie in the wavelength of visible light. The usefulness of the instrument can be increased simply by various methods of illumination. Dark background illumination and the use of fluorescent stains with a suitable source of light, are both important. Modifications of the optical microscope include stereoscopic vision, zoom lenses, upside down microscopes, so that substances floating in media can be examined in a chamber. Microscopes mounted to allow their use for various operative procedures particularly inside the ear are associated with opthalmoscopes. The resolving power of microscopes is vastly increased in the electron microscope and the scanning electron microscopes which use beams of electrons bent by electromagnetic fields instead of light bent by lenses. Electron microscopy is the limitation of all microscopy in that the structure has to be stained to make it opaque to electrons and it has to be cut to a suitably thin section. The scanning electron microscope and surface etching processes overcome this problem to a certain extent. Associated with microscopy is a large amount of ancillary equipment for cutting and preparing sections.

■ **Needleless injector**

A method for injecting without using a needle. The drug to be injected is squirted at an extremely high pressure through a fine nozzle. The pressure is high enough to penetrate the skin and carry the drug into the deeper tissues.

▲● **Oscillograph**

Direct writing and recording. A device for producing a permanent record of the variation, usually with time, of a property to be measured.

▲● **Oscilloscope**

A device for displaying on the screen of a cathode-ray tube a trace representing the variation, usually with time, of a particular property to be measured. Multiple channel oscilloscope permits the simultaneous recording of a number of different properties. Variable persistence oscilloscope allows the duration of the display on the screen, after the event, to be varied.

▲ Osmometer

Instrument for measuring concentration of solutes. Membrane osmometers give faster results than ultracentrifuges and can give molecular weights for nucleic acids, serum albumin, polypeptides, and polysaccharides etc.

■ Oxygenator

Device for removing CO_2 from live blood and replenishing its oxygen. In *disk* oxygenators rotating disks lift blood film into O_2 environment; need small priming blood volume; some are disposable and cheap. *Drum* oxygenators worked on the same principle but have been ousted by the more efficient disk machines. In *screen* oxygenators blood is poured in a film down vertical screens or meshes; designed to reduce hemolysis caused by rotating disks; needs big priming volume. *Bubble* oxygenators rely on rising mass of oxygen bubbles in a column of blood; needs little priming blood but can damage blood by denaturing protein. All carry risk of letting O_2 into bloodstream. *Membrane* oxygenators, still in the experimental stage, in which blood and gases are separated by a membrane, offer many advantages— low prime, little blood damage, no protein denaturing.

■ Pacemaker

Driven by battery, nuclear power, induction coil, piezoelectricity, electrolytically, or by subcutaneous photoelectric cell. Implantable pacemakers may operate on a fixed rate (with 2 speeds changed by passing a magnet over the skin to work a magnetic switch), or on demand (when the patient's own conductivity fails) or on an atrial trigger, picking up the natural pulse and amplifying it before delivering it back to the heart. The pulse from all pacemakers is usually about 2 volts and lasts 2 milliseconds; the wave form is square. An external pacemaker, used in emergency and temporary situations, works via a catheter passing along a vein into the right ventricle.

▲ pH electrodes

Electrode consisting of two cells:

1. Thin glass bulb containing known concentration of HCl into which dips a silver wire coated with silver chloride, making a half cell of silver/silver chloride/HCl whose characteristics are accurately known at a given temperature. When immersed in a solution whose pH is unknown a potential proportional to pH is produced.

2. Reference calomel (= Mercurous chloride) electrode whose inner tube contains mercury, calomel, KCl paste, and wire contact through glass to outer tube; this contains saturated KCl, which makes contact through plug with solution whose pH is to be measured. Current passed in proportion to pH.

▲ Phonocardiograph (PKG)

Microphone-amplifier-recorder system to monitor heart sounds. Can also be used to monitor sounds from esophagus.

▲ Photoelectric specific gravity measurer

Device for measuring the specific gravity of very small volumes of physiological fluids. A plummet of precisely known density is sunk in the fluid and a photocell measures its position with high accuracy.

▲ Photomicrography

Photography through a microscope. Provides an objective record of histology sections, bacteriology studies, and so on.

▲ **Platelet aggregation meter**

Device for measuring the aggregation of blood platelets in the presence of ATP; degree of aggregation is shown by decrease in light absorption of sample. This aggregation is sometimes a better measure of clotting activity than measurement of prothrombin time, the other common test.

▲● **Plethysmograph**

An instrument designed for measuring volume as a method of estimating regional blood flow. For example, a patient's arm can be placed in a container, the residual volume of which can be accurately measured in order to record changes in blood volume following the administration of drugs etc.

■ **Portable operating theater**

Can be used for emergencies such as earthquakes, in war time and for temporary use in hospitals where the theaters are out of use. Consists of plastic air-conditioned tent with theater services.

▲● **Pressure transducer**

Slim low-deformation pressure sensors for incorporation in bandages or plasters to measure pressure without interfering with procedure.

■ **Pressure wave apparatus**

Device for massaging patient by using inflatable cuffs or belts. The pressure waveform is variable so as to control the type and degree of massage.

■ **Prosthetic limbs**

Many versions varying from simple pegleg to sophisticated electromechanical artificial hands triggered by electromyograph impulses. Most commonly used are hooklike devices.

▲● **Pulmonary function analyzer**

Uses radioactive gas inhalation or intravenous gas injection of radioactive xenon, and scans chest with twelve detector system to see distribution of radioactivity—thus revealing dead or stagnant areas.

▲ **Pulse rate meter**

Detector that clips on fingers or thumb and senses pulse either through expansion or by shining light through finger onto cadmium sulphide photocell. Can be set to trigger light, alarm, noise, or counter.

■ **Pumps**

Those used in medicine must meet stringent tests for accuracy and gentleness—especially those that handle blood. Common types are:

Peristaltic: A series of metal rods press down on a tube and then rise in succession, describing a moving sine wave.

Roller and tube: A roller massages fluid through a tube.

Syringe: A plunger displaces fluid through an outlet valve and then draws a fresh charge through an inlet valve.

Valve: Many pumps have valves that mimic human ventricular action.

Fluid-logic: Fluid-logic devices are being intensively researched; they offer such possibilities as automatic and highly responsive control, lack of moving parts, lack of blood-destructive forces.

One experimental pump involves rhythmically and partially compressing a tube at two adjacent sites slightly out of phase.

▲ **Pyrolyzer**

Device for identifying nonvolatile organic compounds such as steroids and polymers by decomposing them at high temperatures. It is vital for the reaction zone to be maintained at precise and constant temperature and free of contaminants and unpyrolized samples.

● **Radiation monitor**

Dose rate meter using built-in Geiger Muller counter. Can be set to give audible warning when given level is reached. Can also be used in placental localization. Blood flows slowly through placenta and pools in sinusoids, therefore scanning picks up maximum intensity over placenta.

▲● **Radioautograph**

Scanning scintillation camera (digital autofluoroscope) with a detector mosaic of 294 small thallium-activated sodium-iodide crystals. In front of the crystals is a multiple channel collimator (up to 3 ins. thick). Crystals are optically connected to 35 photomultiplier tubes. Phototubes feed amplifier which feeds digital computer. Can be set to scan whole or part of body and reveal abnormalities in metabolism and blood-flow.

● **Radiocardiography**

10 millicurie of barium 137 is injected into subclavian vein. Counters over ventricles and the aorta follow its passage and provide a timing. Used with phonocardiograph and EKG. Can help diagnosis. (*See also* Renogram.)

● **Radio pill (Endoradiosonde)**

Small, sealed transmitter that, when swallowed, transmits physiological data (temperature, pH, pressure). Mercury-battery powered, it can be recovered and re-used. Best reception is given by a 3-directional belt antenna linked to chart recorder. Intracranial pressure can also be measured using a radio pill.

■ **Radiotherapy simulator**

It is important to work out the dosage of irradiation very accurately. This can be done with a simulator in which, apart from the substitution of a "phantom" for the patient (or the relevant form of him) all conditions are as they will be during therapy.

● **Rapid mass spectrometer**

A time-of-flight mass spectrometer capable of taking measurements in less than 10 μ seconds. Used for determining instantly the exact composition of a gas, e.g. an anesthetic. The principle is to ionize gases or vapors and to accelerate the ions along a field-free drift tube. The ions separate into bunches with velocities inversely proportional to the mass of the particular ion; thus the low mass ions arrive at the end of the drift tube earlier than the high mass, producing a spectrum at a suitable practical detector.

▲● **Renogram**

System for radio-isotope examination of the kidney following injection of iodine-131-labeled hippuran. Scintillation counters over kidneys connected to ratemeters and pen recorders reveal rate of excretion (kidney function).

▲ **Respiratory flow (Measuring instruments)**

Many simple devices (propellors, bellows, reservoir bag), are available to measure gas flow either during anesthesia or in the intact subject. Most are coupled to artificial ventilators to record the actual output of the ventilator, as opposed to the theoretical output.

▲ **Respiration monitor**

Device used for checking respiratory function during anesthesia; records peak flow, tidal volume, minute volume and rate.

■ **Ripple beds**

Alternating pressure pads to prevent bedsores. Special pads to go under lower sheet consisting of multiple air chambers alternately inflated to move weight bearing from place to place. Actuated either by out of phase pumps or by flip-flop valves.

▲ **Scintillation detector**

A device for detecting the emission of α and β particles arising from the decay of atoms of a radioactive substance. The collision of the particle with the detector is indicated by a flash of light. (*See also* Radioautograph.)

■ **Short-wave diathermy**

Physiotherapy machines that use radio frequency (just over 11-meter wavelength) waves to warm tissues in depth.

■ **Sinusoidal electrostimulator**

Used by physiotherapists to stimulate nerves, muscle, and skin to promote circulatory improvement.

▲ **Spectroscope**

An instrument for resolving electromagnetic radiation (usually visible light) into its component wavelengths for the purpose of identifying the element or elements from which it is derived.

In an absorption spectrometer particular wavelengths from a polychromatic source are absorbed by excited atoms of the element to be analyzed. Each element has its characteristic pattern of absorption.

▲ **Sphygmomanometer**

Mercury manometer connected to a cuff around the patient's arm to record his blood pressure. The pressure (recorded in the column of mercury) is raised until the vessels are completely occluded; then it is slowly lowered until the arterial blood pressure can just separate the walls of the vessel allowing them to fall together again with an audible sound. Further reduction in pressure results in an increase in sound due to the increasing excursion of the vessel walls until silence indicates that diastolic blood pressure is now enough to prevent the vessel walls from coming into contact.

■ **Sterile air flow cabinet**

Many medical processes such as preparing homograft valves require a local sterile environment, usually obtained by working in a closed container with a laminar of bacterially filtered air, often with ultraviolet light.

■ **Sterilizers**

Materials that cannot be heated (*see* Autoclave) must be chemically sterilized. The same is true in the sterilization of biological grafts. Ethylene-oxide gas and betapropreolactone are suitable agents. Both are poisonous and must be removed before use—ethylene oxide in a vacuum, betapropreolactone by reaction with pure water.

● **Stroboscope**

A device for apparently arresting motion either by a regular series of flashes of light synchronous with the motion or by a similar regular interruption of the light reflected from the object under observation.

▲ **Sudorimeter**

A small chamber sealed by being held against the skin. A humidity-measuring device within the chamber measures the degree of sweating. Helps anestheticians to check a patient's progress during anesthesia.

▲● **Thermocouple**

A junction between two dissimilar metals forming part of an electric circuit. If the junction is maintained at a temperature different from the remainder of the circuit a potential difference will be produced across the junction which can be used to measure the temperature.

▲● **Thermograph**

Infrared camera using fast film that can detect 0.1°c differences. Can spot early breast cancer and locate sites where arterial blood flow is poor.

▲● Thermodilution cardiac output computer

Instrument that measures temperature rise in aorta downstream from an injection of warm saline at known temperature. Temperature change depends on cardiac output.

■ Thermoelectric cooling system

System for producing localized cold source using the Peltier effect. (A thermocouple when it has a current run through it has a cold end and a hot end. If the "hot" end is cooled enough, the cold end gets really cold.) Temperatures of $-25°c$ can easily be obtained. Though thermodynamically inefficient (and therefore expensive) it has the great advantage of localization.

■ Ultrasonic cleanser

Wherever possible, apparatus used for injection or for connection to a patient should be disposable. Where this is not possible, foreign material can be removed by using a special detergent, agitated by ultrasound in order to vibrate off foreign material.

■● Ultrasound image converter

Greater sensitivity to reduce risk of tissue damage. Piezoelectric plate is used to pick up impinging ultrasound which is then amplified through electron multiplier and displayed on conventional T.V.

Acknowledgments

The author expresses his profound gratitude to the following people and organizations, each of whom in some way made possible this book and the work it describes:

Medical colleagues Dr. Eunice Lockey, Sir T. Holmes Sellors, Mr. Donald Ross, Dr. Mark Patterson, Dr. Norman Longden Jones, Professor Denis Melrose, Dr. Nora Burns, Prof. E. C. Amoroso, Mr. John Charnley, Dr. Frank Beswick, Dr. L. C. Thomas, Dr. P. Pampiglione, Dr. Ian Hopkinson, Dr. Gordon Hall, Prof. J. Bishop, Dr. John Jackson, Dr. Dennis Deuchar, Dr. Ray Gosling and countless research fellows, helpers and friends.

Engineering colleagues Mr. R. M. Bass, Sir George Dowty, Mr. J. Hunt, Dr. D. Denny, G. D. Allen and P. Burgess Allen, Mr. Steele, Mr. I. Horn, Mr. J. Dobbie, Mr. P. Stiles, Mr. M. Laxton, Mr. Henry Light, Mr. S. W. Sargent, Mr. P. Hills.

Technicians B. Lewis, C. Gilmore, J. Manders, N. Nizrani, A. K. Kamalagharan, J. Boyd, J. Nixon, G. Williams, and B. Richards.

Firms and organizations The British National Health Service, the British Heart Foundation, the Institute of Cardiology, Boehringer Ingelheim, Beecham Research Laboratories, Chemical Defence Experimental Establishment, Porton Down, Allen Die & Tool Co., Barr & Stroud, Dowty Organisation, Electronic Switchgear Ltd., Vickers Research, Medelec, Scotland Yard Forensic Laboratory, I.B.M. U.K., Ltd.

Suggested Reading

If this book has kindled your interest in physiology, you will find excellent general reviews in *The Human Body* by C. H. Best and N. B. Taylor, Chapman and Hall (London, 1966) Holt Rinehart and Winston (New York, 1966) and its bigger brother *The Physiological Basis of Medical Practice* edited by Best and Taylor, E. and S. Livingstone (Edinburgh and London, 1967) Williams and Wilkins (Baltimore 8th Ed., 1966). William F. Ganong's *Review of Medical Physiology*, Lange Medical Publications (California, 1967) Blackwell Scientific Publications (Oxford, 1967) is thorough, up-to-date and well illustrated. *Clinical Physiology* edited by E. J. M. Campbell, C. J. Dickenson, and J. D. H. Slater, Blackwell Scientific Publications (Oxford, 1968) F. A. Davis and Co. (Philadelphia, 1968) is also of fundamental interest and importance. The mysteries of EEG interpretation are made clear in *The EEG in Clinical Practice* by J. P. Laidlaw and J. B. Stanton,

E. and S. Livingstone (Edinburgh and London, 1966) Williams and Wilkins (Baltimore, 1966), which prints a number of recordings together with detailed diagnoses. One of the best and most provocative books on EKGs is *Introduction to Electrocardiography* by L. Schamroth, Blackwell Scientific Publications (Oxford 3rd Ed., 1966) F. A. Davis and Co. (Philadelphia, 1966). The best guides to chemical measurement in medicine are (in my experience) the explanatory handbooks put out by the manufacturers of the actual machines. *Computers in the Service of Medicine* edited by G. McLachlan and R. A. Shegog, Oxford University Press (London and New York, 1968) is a good state-of-the art report; its final chapters provide an interesting and most readable glimpse of the possible future. *Towards a Hospital Computer Service*, a handbook from the United Birmingham Hospitals (England), describes one system in exhaustive detail, and articles in the *Journal of the American Medical Association* (Vol 205, numbers 5, 9, and 12 and Vol 206, number 2) offer fascinating glimpses of further computer applications. I have found *Biomedical Engineering* (a monthly journal published from 9 Gough Square, London, E.C.4, and 3701 Connecticut Avenue NW, Washington DC 20008) of enormous value—both while writing this book and in professional life; it has all the trade news as well as several articles on fundamentals in each issue. Books of general interest close to the themes raised by this volume include my own *Spare-Part Surgery*, to which this is the sequel, *The Biological Time Bomb* by Gordon Rattray Taylor, Thames and Hudson (London, 1968) New American Library (New York, 1968), *An Inquiry Concerning Growth, Disease and Ageing* by Dr. Philip Burch, Oliver and Boyd (London, 1968), and—as an insight into the actual process of science—*The Double Helix* by James Watson, Weidenfeld and Nicolson (London, 1968) Atheneum (New York, 1968).

Picture Credits

8 Photo Ken Coton © Aldus Books, courtesy Dr. D. E. Nicholson, University of Leeds, England and Koch-Light Laboratories Ltd., Colnbrook, England: 13 (Top) Sidney Woods; (Bottom) Photo Ken Moreman, A.I.I.P., F.R.P.S.: 24 Photo Roger Hyde © Aldus Books, courtesy Specialised Laboratory Equipment, Croydon, England: 26 after Sir John Eccles, © January, 1965, *Scientific American*, Inc. All rights reserved: 32 Photo Roger Hyde © Aldus Books, courtesy Specialised Laboratory Equipment, Croydon, England: 36 Photo Professor H. E. Huxley; Diagrams after H. E. Huxley, *The Mechanism of Muscular Contraction*, © December 1965, *Scientific American*, Inc. All rights reserved: 39 Photo Donald B. Longmore: 44 Photo Ken Moreman, A.I.I.P., F.R.P.S.: 52 (Bottom) Sidney Woods: 53, 56, 61 Photos Donald B. Longmore: 64 Photos Roger Hyde © Aldus Books, courtesy Technicon Instrument Co. Ltd., Chertsey, England:

188

Index

192

phagocytic vesicles, 15
phonocardiograph (PKG), 69, 84, 87, 91
phospholipids, 15-6, 17
phrenic nerve, 28
pinocytic vesicles, 15
plasma, 57, 58, 65, 66, 147
PO₂: alveolar, 100; arterial, 48; definition of, 47-8; measurement of 49-51, 50, 52; of blood, 47-51, 47, 52, 58, 87, 94-5; venous, 47, 48, 100
polycarbonate, 103
polydimethylsiloxane, 93, 100, 102, 117
polymerization of sugar molecules in blood, 156, 158
polymer membranes, breathability of various, 98
polythene tent isolator, 114, 115
potassium, 20, 27, 27, 46, 52, 52, 67, 91
PQRST complex, 42, 42
profile: biochemical, 166-7; surgical, 140; therapeutic, 140
proportioning pump: in AutoAnalyzer, 62, 64; in dialyzate automixer, 108-110, 115
pulmonary: artery, 77, 79, 87, 88, 89; edema, see edema; valve, 79, 84, 88; valve stenosis, 89 vein, 77, 79
punch cards: in hospital organization, 126-138, 129, 131, 133, 135, 137
P wave, 41, 43

QRS complex, 41-2, 43
QRST complex, 43

radio pill, 75, 75
reflection photometer, 49-51, 52
respiratory tests, 79-83
reserve volume, 79
residual volume, 80-1
ribosome, 12
Royal Postgraduate Medical School, London, 101, 103-4
R waves, 43

sarcolemma, 35
septal defects, see heart
scintillation counter, 73, 83

silicone rubber, see membrane
sinu-atrial (SA) node, 38, 43
sodium, 16, 18, 20, 27-8, 27, 52, 52, 67, 91, 108-9
sodium/potassium ion pump, 17, 27-8, 27, 91
spectrophotometry, 51-54, 63
spectrum of machines, 161, 163, 163
spirometer, 79-80, 81, 82, 85, 91
stenosis, 79, 87; see also mitral valve and pulmonary
sterile aircurtaining techniques, 112, 114-5
superior vena cava, 46, 87
surfactants, 105

Technicon AutoAnalyzer, 62-3, 64
therapeutic: effects, 141; machines, 93-119, 93, 159; profiles, see profile
therapy, 23, 25, 49, 84, 110, 142, 142, 147, 159-61, 166; definition of, 160
thyroid deficiency, 142
tidal volume, 79, 82
tricuspid valve, 87, 89, 90
T wave, 41, 43

ureters, 71-2
urine, 45, 57, 71, 91; normal pH of, 56; analysis of, 62

valves: heart see heart
V electrodes, 41
venous: pressure, 91, 95 pulses, 84
ventricular: muscle, 38, 41; pressure, 89; septal defect, 88; septum, 38
Vickers Multichannel 300, 63, 65, 66-7, 133, 137
vital capacity, 79, 81-2, 85, 91
vitreous humor, 32
V leads, 39, 41

wedge-streamlining effect, 76, 77, 80

X rays, 10, 46, 73, 74, 76, 78, 82, 83, 87, 88, 91, 118, 124, 126, 127, 138, 150